MY AMAZING JOURNEY with THE DIVINE

*A Reiki Energy Healer's
Firsthand Experience with
Miracles in Healings*

BEVERLY A. POKORSKI

Library of Congress Control Number: 2018967578

ISBN: 978-0-9977477-3-7

First Printing: January, 2019

Imprint: 102nd Place, LLC
         Scottsdale, AZ

Printed in the United States of America

DISCLAIMER

This book and the methods described in this book are **NOT** intended as a substitute for professional advice, diagnosis, or treatment. Always seek advice from a licensed medical professional for any physical, mental, psychological or emotional disorder. This book is not intended to diagnose, treat or cure any disease or disorder. Significant changes in your health or health regime should be discussed with your health care provider. The opinions, advice and recommendations in this book are intended for a wide audience of people and are not tailored or specific to any individual needs or health conditions. The authors and publishers of this book make no warranty, representation, or guarantee regarding the practices or advice given in this book, nor do they assume any liability whatsoever arising out of your use of any information or treatments referenced in this book. The authors and publishers of this book are not responsible for any harm or injuries that you might incur as a result of following the advice in this book. To protect client privacy, the names have been changed.

Dedication

"Do this in memory of me."

(Luke 22:19)

I dedicate this book to the Miraculous Healing Powers of The Divine, from Whom Jesus, His Miracles, Blessed Mother Mary, Her Miracles, the Angels, Mother Kwan Yin and all the Ascended Masters, Saints, our Spirit and Reiki Guides and their Miracles come, along with the Highest and Greatest Good.

I am writing this book in the hope that you will see, as I have been shown, that there is a Higher Power. A Power that is Divine, Magnificent, Benevolent, All Powerful and All Knowing. This Power, I call God. He is Perfect, Unconditional Love, and is always there for each and every one of us. We are all connected to Him and to each other. We are all Energy Beings living in a physical body, sharing human experiences together for the growth and evolution of our Souls.

I am writing this book to tell Grace's story and that of many others who have been Saved, Healed and Touched by Divine Intervention.

I am writing this book to share with you my most Amazing Journey in Energy Healing . . . a Journey truly with The Divine.

I would like to especially thank God, His Son, Jesus, the Blessed Mother Mary, Saint Joseph, Archangels Michael, Raphael, and all of God's Divine Angels, Mother Kwan Yin and all the Ascended Masters, Saints, Spirit Guides, and Loved Ones who are with me. They surround me and my clients, during each and every Healing Session, with God's Divine Love and Light. I would also like to thank all of those who invited me to be a part of their most Amazing Journeys. To all of You, with love, gratitude, humility and respect, I dedicate this book.

CONTENTS

FOREWORD

It amazes me when one of your clients that you meet for the first time and you sense this person is a true healer but does not know it yet; that is what I felt when I first met Beverly.

She did not know what energy healing was but every time we had a session, she felt tingling and other sensations throughout her body. She would experience visions, hearing voiceless voices and other intuitive abilities. I knew it was a matter of time when I would be able to mention her learning energy healing.

As the old saying goes, "When the student is ready, the teacher appears." That time finally came, and I taught her self-healing. Her abilities began advancing overnight and Beverly had the ability to do distant healing beyond any other person I had trained including myself. I then began referring cancer clients to her and the results were amazing! Her distant healing created miracles! Beverly's abilities were truly angelic! I was proud beyond words!

When I need healing, I would ask Beverly. Her healing is pure and always coming from unconditional love and light. I know in my heart that her angels are always guiding and helping her with her abilities. In my book, I mention that as you enter into the world of energy healing, see within yourself that stable center, that perfect seed, the perfection, your potential. Allow yourself to move inward to the center and the core of your being. At the core of your very being, there is a diamond of perfection. The universal light, the light of love, is within you. Beverly is truly a diamond of perfection.

I thank God, every day for the day I met Beverly! Our world needs more healers and the angelic realm, and God I know are proud to have this one on their side!

Barbara E. Savin, *Author of "Gentle Energy Touch, The Beginner's Guide to Hands-On Healing," Master Energy Healing Specialist, Clinical & Medical Hypnotherapist, Reiki Master/Teacher, Life Coach Consultant and Spiritual Teacher.*

INTRODUCTION

For the better part of my adult life, I could and would describe myself as a linear thinker. The left side of my brain was the dominant side, where math, science and logic resided. I excelled in them, was very comfortable with them and even studied medicine later in life.

I find it so ironic that I have actually written a book, since I spent the entire part of my college career searching out courses that did not require me to write even a single paper!

I have been very Blessed with these intellectual abilities. They have served me well and continue to do so.

Later in life, I came to realize the Blessings of God's Spiritual Gifts of Divine Healing, connection and intuition.

They serve my clients and myself in Amazing and Wondrous ways!!!

Until 2009, I, like many others, was unfamiliar with Reiki Energy Healing. That was when I found my mentor and Healer, Barbara Savin.

Reiki is a Japanese word that means God's (Rei) Life Force (ki). This is the Universal Life Force or Divine Energy that is transferred from God to my clients, using me as a conduit or vessel.

As my mentor Barbara Savin would say, "I am just the plug," much like when your radio, television set or computer is plugged in and turned on. We cannot see the radio or television waves as they are being sent, but we can hear them and view our TV and computer screens when we plug them in and turn them on. I and my clients have seen and felt God's Magnificent Energy as it was being transferred from Him through me to them. The results of His Miraculous Healings are tangible, true, observable and documented.

Many great pioneers of the 20th century were fascinated with the study of energy: Albert Einstein, Nicolas Tesla and Madame Curie, just to name a few.

I personally love this quote by Albert Einstein,

"There are only two ways to live your life: as though nothing is a miracle, or as though everything is a miracle."

I prefer to look at this wonderful and sometimes messy life as a Miracle! I look at the pure and precious, innocent babies, and all the joy that they bring into our lives.

I see the brilliance and feel the warmth of the sun, shining on us and sustaining our lives.

I see the stars and the moon lighting up the night sky.

I see, hear and feel the oceans, giving us beauty, recreation, peace and Healing.

I see the whales, the dolphins and the birds.

I see all of God's Creation and I ask myself; How could you possibly not believe in Miracles?!!!

Reiki Energy Healing is Spiritually Guided and Directed by God. His Energy flows through me from my head into my hands, to be exchanged with my clients.

Somehow, I am able to bring my client's energy to me and feel their energy field as if they were lying on my Healing table in person.

This brings to mind a conversation that I just had with my son about how people can now work remotely via their computers. They can communicate with each other instantaneously through written words and live videos. They do this from different locations, but their computers bring them face to face with each other. This is probably the best analogy I can think of to explain my ability to do this with other people's energy fields.

We still do not understand enough about quantum physics to be able to explain this scientifically or why distance Healing is more powerful than an in-person Healing. It seems to be akin to separate waves that eventually converge into one concentrated wave over distance, that magnifies their energies.

I think this might explain why Prayer Healings

are so powerful because all of the separate energies and intentions of the people who are praying all converge to focus on the recipient of their Prayers.

On becoming a Master Reiki Healer, I have been very Blessed with an Amazing ability to connect with The Divine. I am in awe of His Magnificence, Power, Benevolence, Love and Grace.

I believe that we all have this ability to connect with our Divine Source because we are all inherently connected to Him and to each other.

I also believe that Healers are born with the ability to Heal and eventually realize and manifest this Gift.

Before we are born, we work with our Spirit Guides and Angels to choose certain lessons that our Souls would like to work on, here on this earth. Hopefully, we can learn and perfect these lessons during our short lifetimes here. We each have a Soul purpose that we have come here to fulfill; a destiny.

My destiny was to be a Healer.

I believe it was also to teach about God's Existence, Benevolence, Power, Grace and Unconditional Love for us.

People often ask me how I manifest this Connection or Gift. First of all, my mentor Barbara Savin did a tremendous job of attuning me to God's Energy!

Attunement is when a Master Reiki teacher channels and transfers God's Energy to the student. This results in opening up the crown, heart and palm chakras, creating a special connection between the student and God's Life Force (Reiki).

There is a Christ Consciousness of perfect Love that a Healer connects with and brings their clients into, in order for them to be Healed.

(Chakras are the main centers of Spiritual power within the human body through which Energy flows.)

This attunement is a very critical part of a Reiki Healer's ability to connect with and transfer God's Energy to their clients.

After my attunement occurred, my answer is that I show up, I ask with a strong will and direct intent, and I Believe. Believing is the most important part. I guess the believing part seems to be the hardest part for most people because it involves something that cannot be adequately understood and explained yet by the scientific community; in other words, it requires Faith! Faith on the part of the Healer and, as I have observed, Faith on the part of the client, even though God's Magnificent Energy can penetrate the strongest barrier. But the results of His Love in His Healings can indeed be tangibly measured! Undeniable and True.

This ability to connect with The Divine did not come easily as I had to overcome great challenges to get there. This difficult path to Enlightenment is not unusual for Healers to have to traverse. It led me to The One Who is Always there for us, especially when all else fails.

Please join me as I invite you to share with me my most Amazing Journey with The Divine.

Beverly

MY STORY

Through pain, I found compassion.
Through weakness, I found strength.
Through hurt, I found forgiveness.
Through heartbreak, I found help.
Through help I found love.
Through love, I found hope.
Through hope, I found faith.
Through faith, I found Miracles.
Through Miracles, I found God.

Beverly A. Pokorski

"But he knows the way that I take; when he has tested me, I will come forth as gold." (Job 23:10)

It all started in earnest in the spring of 2009. In retrospect, I think I was being prepared for this Journey a long time before then, very slowly, with psychic experiences with loved ones that had passed over. Incredible things would happen to me, my loved ones and my possessions.

Some of the first psychic experiences that I remember happening took place immediately after my Grandfather's passing.

After my Grandfather's funeral, appliances would turn on and off by themselves, the volume on the TV would go up and down by itself, and dishes would seem to get pulled out of my hands while I would unload the dishwasher. Of course, the scientist in me then tried to logically explain all of these strange occurrences.

My Grandfather had also made his presence known to his beloved wee little relatives. It had been reported that he would tickle them in their beds and talk to them on their toy phones. When their parents would hear them giggling like crazy, they would run up to their room to see what was going on and that is what they were told. These strange happenings continued for a month after my grandfather's death. Then on the first month anniversary of his passing, I found a fine, thin gold chain in my drawer that previously was hopelessly entangled with hundreds of knots. That morning, I opened the drawer and it was laid out perfectly straight, without a single knot! When my husband came home that evening, I thanked him for detangling my chain and asked him when he had done that for me. He said that he had no idea what I was talking about. So, I took him over to the drawer where I had found the detangled gold chain and opened it. He turned ghostly white and said that he had tried but had given up because it was impossibly tangled. He was visibly shaken! That was the final incidence with my grandfather's Spirit after he had passed.

Despite all the scientific explanations that I kept coming up with to explain all the unusual events that had been taking place over that past month, this last one was truly unexplainable, at least according to the earthly world that we live in.

The next large group of psychic experiences occurred immediately after my Mother passed. We flew cross country from Los Angeles to New York to attend her funeral and settle her affairs. I had called my brother in New York, who was with my Mom as she was passing, to inform him that we were leaving for the airport. When he answered, he told me that my dear, beloved Mother had just taken her last breath. Needless to say, I was devastated, not only that she had passed but that I could not have been there with her when she did.

On the red-eye flight back to my childhood home, I witnessed something very beautiful. There was a group of stars in the sky, right outside the window of our plane. They were outlined in the shape of a heart. A shooting star appeared and shot right through the center of that heart of stars.

I have never seen a shooting star either before or after that beautiful display.

When we arrived in New York, I had understandably not slept and was up all-night feeling very distraught and upset. My brother met us at the airport and commented on how bedraggled I looked. I felt even worse. We proceeded to go on to our Mother's home to freshen up for the long day ahead. As soon as we entered her home, both my husband and I felt this extreme sense of joy and giddiness bubbling up from and filling the inside of our chests, filling our hearts. I knew that we were feeling my Mom's energy and that she was filled with joy and in a Magnificent Place.

We then checked into our hotel for the arduous task of preparing for my Mother's funeral. On the morning of the funeral, we heard the piano in the dining room playing at 6:00 a.m. The room was scheduled to open for breakfast every morning at 8:00 a.m. So, I asked the owner, who I had become friends with from many previous stays, if she was playing the piano that morning. She said "no." The room had been locked until 8:00 a.m. for breakfast, as it always had been. (It is interesting to note that my parents bought a beautiful piano for me when I was a child. They used to love to sit in our living room and listen to me while I played.)

Not only that, but as we were getting ready for the funeral, all the electricity went out in our suite, only ours!

After the funeral, we brought a dear loved one back to our suite to spend the night. Both our loved one and I started noticing a beautiful white light coming into our room from the window. Then we noticed little white lights all over the ceiling that looked like little stars. My loved one reported seeing a vision of the Blessed Mother Mary. I felt a profound sense of joy, peace and comfort.

The day after my Mother's funeral, my dearest friend noticed a beautiful white light emanating from the center of a decorative tree in the corner of her dining room. She took notice of it after she heard my Mother's voice calling to her from that room, which was the next room directly behind her. She turned around as she heard my Mother's voice coming from the light and called out my Mom's name in shock, with a question in her voice. The voice told my friend that a dear loved one of my Mom's was going to love my friend's home. My Mother used her special nickname for our loved one, which my friend could not have known. We were all scheduled to visit with my friend that very same evening in her home.

This same very dear friend had a beautiful vision of my Mom and Dad shortly after my Mother passed. They were both together in a beautiful verdant valley. She described everything about my Dad in such accurate detail, things she did not know about him when he was alive. The way he sat with my Mom on the ground with his ankles crossed, the way he rolled up his shirt sleeves and the pocket where he kept his cigarettes. I knew then that they were together again after a decade of being apart, happily reunited.

When we arrived back home in L.A., we noticed that the roses that were cut from our garden and placed in a vase inside our home before we left for the funeral were quite dried and shriveled up when we got back. I commented to my husband that we needed to replace them with fresh ones. The next morning when I awoke, I noticed that several of the roses in the center of the dead bouquet were alive and full of dew! Neither my husband nor I had touched them or replaced them yet!

Months after my Mom's passing, I had a vision of her when I was lying in bed with terrible back pain. The pain was so bad that I could not even get out of bed by myself! (I remember my husband having to pull me straight down off of the bed because I could not bend my back to sit up.) She was standing in the doorway of my bedroom, looking at me with a very concerned expression on her face. She appeared to be biting her fingernails. Then she faded away. At times, I would smell her perfume enveloping me.

Every night for a year, as soon as I got settled into bed, my phone would ding just once. A month after my Mom's passing, during my son's high school graduation party, the light fixture above our kitchen breakfast table started flickering so badly above us that my guests were starting to notice and look very uncomfortable. This phenomenon only happened on that very special day.

I remember a particularly sad day, when I was missing my Mom tremendously. I was driving alone in my car and the song that was popular when she got sick came on the radio. The song was called *"My Heart Will Go On"* from the movie *"Titanic."* It was my song to her. With tears in my eyes, I tried to push a CD into the slot in the dash of my car in order to replay the song, but it kept pushing back out against me over and over again. Never happened before or since!

So, I guess all along, I did have psychic abilities and connections, but little did I know that they would develop into the Healing Gift that I have received.

Now, we fast forward to 2009. It was smack in the middle of government incentives for first-time home buyers. I was wanting to move down to my favorite town on the ocean and I thought that I had found the perfect home.

But, not so fast! Nothing I could do would make the seller sell me that house. My realtor said that he had seen nothing like it in the 50 years that he was in the business. I had so many appointments to show the house that I needed to sell that it literally was insane! Little did I know then that my current home where I now live on the ocean, was the dream home that was waiting for me. But . . . it was not the home I was so desperately trying to buy.

At the same time, I started to develop a cough from acid reflux, caused by all the stress of the whole experience. I had a throat scope that had two chemicals in it, one of which I was allergic to and the other one was a very harsh chemical used in professional chemical labs for experiments. It was being used as a preservative in the throat numbing cocktail. My throat and esophagus were burnt to the point where I was unable to eat for several months. My doctors could not properly diagnose the problem, so they made matters worse by throwing a very strong anti-anxiety drug at it that has a very long half-life. I lacked the gene necessary to metabolize it, so it kept building up in my body. Needless to say, within two weeks, I found myself in very deep trouble. I pulled my house off the market and gave up on my dream of moving to my favorite town on the ocean.

That is when I found my mentor and Energy Healer, Barbara E. Savin. She literally helped save my life. She was the only one who knew what was wrong. She kept telling my docs that she felt a burn. She was spot on! She even predicted when I would be able to eat again! She was right.

From the very first Energy Healing with Barbara, I could feel God's Energy entering my body from the top of my head. It felt like a tingling, electrical sensation.

On the day before I had to have a test that could have caused me to aspirate a huge amount of barium into my lungs, I scheduled a Healing with Barbara because I was afraid to have that test. I had abruptly stopped the drugs, which was absolutely the wrong thing to do and it could have resulted in seizures. Barbara felt a very powerful Presence behind her during my Healing. She asked who was there and He said Jesus Christ! I now know that He was there to save me from the horrible fate that could have happened the next morning during that test.

It took me several weeks to detox. It definitely was the worst experience of my life, not just physically but mentally and emotionally. Prior to this experience, I would decline even the use of Tylenol unless I was in dire need. I used only natural healing therapies. During the detox period, I could not even get through the reading of a whole sentence because of the resultant brain fog from the detox process. Up until that horrible time, the one thing I could always rely on was my brain's high level of functioning. But my brain and body became totally hijacked by a pharmaceutical drug and the situation was totally beyond my control.

After the detox was completed, I was left with almost unbearable rebound anxiety. Before taking this drug, I had never experienced a panic attack. Afterwards, I experienced many. I remember having a panic attack once that lasted almost twelve hours! There was a point where I did not know if I could go on like that any longer. . . .

But by the Grace of God, I hung in there!

I continued to have weekly Healing sessions with Barbara. They were the only treatments that provided relief from the terrible anxiety that this horrible drug had left me to deal with!

I felt such a wonderful sense of peace and calm during and after each session. Many times, I felt icy cold coming from Barbara's hands through the blankets. She often felt intense heat, while I was simultaneously feeling the cold. Many Divine Beings, Angels, and loved ones were there during my Healing Sessions.

After one of my Healing sessions with Barbara, she described my grandfather to a tee and said he was there with us during my session. He also relayed to Barbara some very comforting personal information to me.

During another session, Barbara had described a very dear friend who had recently passed. She was holding a black briefcase like the one I used in

Phoenix when I was studying naturopathic medicine. I had no idea what she was trying to tell me at the time, but now I know she was telling me that I would eventually study to become an Energy Healer.

I recall a lovely event that happened at the end of another one of my personal Healing Sessions with Barbara. A deceased relative of a friend of mine came to Barbara in a vision with a message for her loved one. She was rocking a baby in her arms and she called herself mother Mary. Barbara relayed this vision to me and asked me if I knew what it meant. I told her that I had no idea what that could mean. I soon forgot about it. The next day, I saw my friend and she immediately told me that her dear loved one had passed. She was very upset, and to make matters worse, she could not attend the funeral because she was not comfortable leaving her baby behind while she traveled to the funeral. I immediately remembered what Barbara had told me and passed this on to my friend. She said that her loved one's name was Mary! This clever spirit used Barbara and me to convey the message to her loved one that it was okay for her to stay at home and take care of her baby. My friend felt very comforted and at peace with her decision then.

The spirit world can be very clever in the ways that they choose to convey their messages to their loved ones here on Earth.

I remember Barbara telling me after one of my

Sessions that "All will be revealed to me." Little did I know then, what was to come! I also remember my last Healing with Barbara right before I moved down to the water where my current dream home awaited me. I had recently started my Distance Healing a few months before. My Mom had come to my Session and told Barbara that "I was doing a very, very good job." Thanks Mom!

At the end of 2011, I started to become interested in self-healing, which Barbara taught me, and in early 2012, I achieved certification to Heal others.

HIS AMAZING GRACE!

"My grace is sufficient for you, for my power is made perfect in weakness." (2 Corinthians 12:9)

Grace's Healings . . . and she lived!

Grace is not her given name. I have chosen to call her Grace because she is alive and well today because of the sheer Grace of God.

Shortly after I became a Master Reiki Energy Healer, I became aware that Grace was in desperate need of a kidney transplant due to complications from diabetes. Her donor also needed help with anxiety because she was very afraid of the surgery and did not tell me at the time of her Healing that donors experience dramatically more pain than the recipients do. I just knew she needed help with the anxiety that she was experiencing while awaiting her surgery.

The stickler was that Grace and her donor lived very far away. I desperately wanted to help them, so I thought that I would try to send God's Healing Energy remotely, also called Distance Healing.

I scheduled a session with Grace's donor and I performed the Healing. It worked! She felt very peaceful, calm, and confident.

(I have found that in order to send Healing, a pure and true desire to help is essential.)

We then agreed to schedule another session immediately after her surgery. As I began her Healing session, I felt a huge throbbing on the side where her kidney would have been. I did not know which kidney was being removed.

After the Healing session, I spoke with her family. They said the surgery was delayed several hours, which meant that I had conducted the Healing right in the middle of her surgery! I then asked them if they knew which kidney had been donated. They said that they did not but that they would find out. When we spoke later, they confirmed what I had felt. It was indeed the side where her kidney had been removed.

The donor then stated that her transplant surgery was successful.

She described feeling a warm sensation traveling through her body and stated that she realized that she was being Healed. She described it as a serene and energizing feeling. The doctors arrived and asked her about her pain. She explained that she felt no pain. She said that she was experiencing only a sensation of pressure. The doctors looked very skeptical, because the donors can expect to experience significant pain. She proceeded to inform them of her Healing during her surgery.

She also reported seeing a deep Purple color behind her eyes when she awoke from the anesthesia, but she felt only pressure, not pain. The surgeon admitted that this was the first patient to report feeling this. She healed without the need for strong pain medication, using only Tylenol.

A few hours after I finished the donor's Healing, I remotely conducted a Session for Grace. Grace described her Healing experience as "incredible."

She was lying in her hospital bed after her kidney transplant. She stated that she felt a calm come over her. She also stated that she saw a stream of Pinkish Purple lights surrounded by Golden shards that came from the sky towards her face and entered her body. She said that she felt strengthened and protected.

Grace's family also reported Grace remembered seeing a Golden, lighted spear or pointed wand that Grace later described to me as resting along her arm down into her hand. I later discovered this pointed wand was a Soul Scepter. It signifies spiritual work and the alignment with Christ-consciousness.

(This Beautiful Healing to Grace also arrived an hour before I actually performed it here on the west coast.)

A little while later, Grace also received a pancreas transplant. I performed another distance Healing on her almost immediately after the transplant. I was perplexed when I felt a lot of heaviness around her heart chakra. It took me quite a while to clear it. When I asked her mother about it, she verified that her daughter was very depressed and would not get out of her hospital bed until after her Healing.

Her mother then told me that after her Healing, Grace jumped up and went to wash her hair, and returned to her normal, happy self. I was still puzzled by this depression, considering that Grace was getting a new lease on life with her new pancreas. A little while later, I got my answer.

During her post-op check-up, her surgeon informed Grace and her mother that the pancreas donor was a young mother who had died in childbirth! So, the heaviness that I felt around Grace's heart at the beginning of her Healing was the donor's, who had just lost her life and her child.

Grace did quite well for several years after her pancreas transplant, but then her body started showing signs of rejection. I did another Distance Healing where she reported feeling a ball of heated Energy in her abdomen that she felt was working to preserve her pancreas.

After quite some time went by, the unthinkable happened. Her pancreas burst along with her colon! She was in ICU literally bleeding to death. No one yet knew what was causing the massive internal bleeding. I started a Healing immediately as soon as I found out. I felt an extreme sense of urgency to begin immediately. I heard thoughts in my head that kept saying repeatedly: "You need to start NOW!" I did not know that she was already in surgery when I started her Healing. This was all being coordinated long distance as her relatives were rushing back to the hospital.

As I began the Healing, I could not feel her energy. That has never happened before. I became very frightened for her. I continued with the Healing and when I reached her heart chakra, I detected a faint energy there. I felt encouraged and kept on going and Praying. When I came near the end of the Healing, where the Healer balances the chakras, I was stunned with the Life Force that was flowing through me into them. It was like being in a very strong wind tunnel with no control on my part. I knew then that she was going to be ok.

(The wind that I felt was God and His Holy Spirit, breathing life back into Grace!)

Immediately after the Healing, I texted the family to tell them that Grace was going to be ok, and at that exact same moment, the surgeon came out and said that she was stable. He stated that the blood they were giving Grace just kept pouring back out of her body. Grace had no blood pressure at all at one point. That is when the surgeon repeatedly said that they were losing her!

I was told that Grace remembered asking God to save her.

I was also told that at Grace's post-op checkup,

her surgeon said that a Miracle had taken place. He suggested that her family consult with their clergy. When Grace explained to him that she had a Healing during her surgery, he paused and thought for a very long time and finally said that he thought he had lost her and that no one has ever survived this kind of ordeal.

. . . and she lived!!!

(This Healing made me feel, as I could only imagine what one must feel like when helping to bring a new life into the world, so joyful and grateful and full of wondrous emotion.)

FAITH'S HEALINGS

"For where two or three gather in my name, there I am with them." (Matthew 18:20)

I call her Faith because of the incredible Faith her family had in God and the giant leap of Faith they took when they entrusted her Healing to a newbie Distance Energy Healer, me!

I was first contacted by Faith's family shortly after I finally found my dream home near the ocean, or I should say it found me. The significance of that distinction will become clearer as these stories continue to unfold.

Faith was diagnosed with multiple myeloma and was suffering from depression, anxiety and lack of appetite.

Faith also developed kidney failure as a complication of her multiple myeloma. This renal condition required Faith to be on dialysis. Her family had asked for a Healing. This Healing was also done over a great distance.

Faith was still acutely aware of her surroundings and reported feeling a wonderful and profound sense of peace during her Healing and afterwards. Her appetite also returned.

A few months later, Faith's family contacted me again. They were extremely distraught because Faith had become critically ill. She not only had multiple myeloma, but now had developed pneumonia and severe sepsis.

Faith now required daily dialysis. Concurrently, *Clostridium difficile* bacteria were present in her intestines. She was subsequently placed on a feeding tube and was generally unaware of her surroundings. She still, to this day, does not remember this particular time in her life. I felt agitation, which always seems to come with these serious situations. I asked that Faith's loved ones please Pray during the Healing that we had scheduled.

At the time of my request to perform a Prayer Healing on Faith, I was not told that she was in multiple organ failure and that her doctor had already prepared her family that it was very unlikely that Faith would survive.

All I felt was a sense of urgency and agitation that always comes to me in these very serious life and death situations. Also, this was the very first Prayer Healing I had performed. I was guided by a thought in my head to suggest this to Faith's family. I am so glad I listened and trusted this Divine Guidance!!!

We scheduled the Healing at an opportune time

when it was unlikely to be interrupted. Everyone started to Pray as soon as I began the Healing. All of Faith's loved ones were in different physical locations from Faith, each other and me. Everyone who Prayed had a significant experience during Faith's Healing.

One of Faith's very close loved ones had gone into a room alone and lit a candle in preparation for Faith's Prayer Healing. During Faith's Healing, her dear loved one reported feeling a total sense of peace and calm. She also described feeling a sensation of White.

(White symbolizes Heaven, purity, faith and spirituality. White is God's Energy.)

Two of Faith's loved ones reported seeing a vision of a cliff above an ocean during the Healing Session. They were both in separate locations from Faith, each other, Faith's other loved ones and me.

When they reported their vision of the cliff above the ocean to me, I thought it might have been the cliff that my Healing table faces. I call it my "Healing Cliff." I took a picture and sent it to them, asking if that is what they saw. They confirmed that was exactly what they saw in their vision!

My Healing table is also looked down upon by a huge Cross that sits atop a church across the ravine from my back deck.

. . . and she lived!!!

Faith is doing well today, in total remission from

her cancer!

Faith now walks a mile a day on the ocean near her home.

Faith's doctors tell her that she is a walking Miracle!!!

I couldn't agree more!!!

(I do not know exactly how a Prayer Healing works, but in my experiences, they seem to magnify God's Healing Energy to the person receiving it.

It is the Love that is expressed for the person and offered up to God in prayer that manifests The Miracles through His Divine Grace.)

HOPE'S HEALING

"May your unfailing love be with us, Lord, even as we put our hope in you." (Psalm 33:22)

"For nothing will be impossible with God." (Luke 1:37)

I call her Hope because she expressed the hope that she would have a nice Healing.

Hope was diagnosed with three malignant tumors in her intestinal tract. Two of the tumors were too large to remove surgically. The doctors had decided to do chemotherapy and radiation in the hope of shrinking the tumors, in order to be able to remove them surgically.

Hope was very anxious about starting the chemotherapy and radiation treatments, so she asked me for a Healing Session before she started her treatments. This Healing was also a Distance Healing. During the Healing, she reported feeling something being threaded down her throat and esophagus to her abdomen. She also reported feeling a sweeping, brushing sensation from her waist down. She said she felt very wonderful and positive, which is how she emotionally and mentally started her treatments.

After the chemotherapy and radiation treatments had shrunk her tumors enough to be operable, Hope scheduled another Healing for the day before her surgery. She told me she hoped to have a nice Healing.

Six weeks had gone by then without any further treatment before her surgery. Her tumors were imaged a week before her surgery to measure the reduction in size from the chemotherapy and radiation treatments that had ended five weeks prior to the imaging. The tumors had only shrunk about one third in size.

At the start of the Healing, Hope had brought in a Prayer cloth that was Blessed. It was a gift to her from a friend.

During the Healing, Hope felt a tugging and pulling sensation and pressure directly on her tumors.

Hope went into surgery the next day. When her surgeon came out after the surgery to report his findings to Hope, he said that he could not find the tumors! All he saw were scalloped edges. The tumors were totally shredded into very thin threads!

He was amazed!!!

Hope had an incredible Healing!

(I do the "Happy Dance "in gratitude whenever I think about Hope's Healing.)

Hope had a successful resection of her colon. All is working well, and she is moving on with her life.

She is doing great!

The results of Hope's two-year post-surgery scans were completely normal!

CHARITY'S HEALINGS
In the Arms of the Angels

"Beyond all these things, put on love, which is the perfect bond of unity." (Colossians 3:14)

I call her Charity because she and her Healings are very dear to my heart.

Charity was diagnosed with Her2 positive breast cancer.

After she was given this shocking news, we set a time for her first Healing Session. This Healing was also conducted over a great distance.

The night that I scheduled Charity's first Healing, I saw a bright yellow object in the shape of a moon, about a third of a moon to be exact, sitting upside down directly below the cross on the stucco wall of the church that faces my Healing table. I could not believe what I was seeing! It was a huge yellow moon, out of the sky, which was physically impossible! So, I went to the adjacent room where my Healing table is and there it was, only it glowed bigger and brighter yellow! By then I was starting to question my cognitive abilities, but I heard a thought in my head that said, "do not be afraid." So, I went back into the other room where I saw it now descending right side up, below and behind the cross until it disappeared below the hill, behind the church and in back of the cross. I had no idea what it meant but when I started Charity's first Healing, the sun was setting through the windows above my French doors that face the cross. It was shining on my face and Healing table, but it was so intense with heat that I thought my hair was going to get singed and I did not look at it. I told myself to keep my eyes closed and go on with the Healing. I believe it was a sign of God's Power, Love and Magnificence and that something Wonderful was about to happen.

Amazingly it did!

I was stunned for days by the Power, Love and Magnificence of the Divine!

(Since writing this, I have been experiencing wonderful visions of the sun also and I believe The Blessed Mother, who moves the sun and the moon, was responsible for the vision of the moon and the heat of the sun as Her Blessing at the start of Charity's first Healing.)

After her very first Healing Session, we spoke immediately, and this is what Charity reported back to me.

During her Healing Session, Charity described feeling energy traveling to the exact physical site of her tumor. Then Charity saw a Spirit appear that looked very much like a Shaman. She asked me if I ever saw my Spirit Guides and if that was what this being could have been. She got the sense that we were both part of a tribal group of women Healers, possibly in a past life.

She reported feeling a very definite and pronounced pulling, tugging, and scooping sensation on her actual tumor. The Spirit actually asked Charity if the tugging was too much for her. She said "no." The Spirit disappeared shortly after.

Charity then reported feeling a sensation in her lymph nodes, especially under the armpit that was on the side of her cancerous tumor. She described feeling a water-like draining sensation, much like water being drained through a sieve.

Before the start of this Healing, Charity told me that she had set her intention to have all cancer cells removed from her lymph nodes.

Charity then reported feeling voices of comfort come to her. She said that they communicated to her not to worry and that they were taking care of her condition.

Charity reported that during her next Healing with me, Angelic-like Beings were present and communicated to her once again to not worry and to trust.

During this Healing, she reported seeing something like large, white, feathery wings that closed over her eyes, that seemed to comfort and shield her. She doesn't remember anything else after this.

She woke up the next day and had her surgery, which was successful.

After her surgery, Charity received the news that her tumor was encapsulated and that her doctors were able to remove it with clear margins. There also was no lymph node involvement reported. Charity said that she believed the Healings she had before her surgery helped to encapsulate the tumor.

Before these Healings, Charity stated that her pathology report from her breast biopsy came back with a Her2 positive cancer result.

After these Healings, Charity received the pathology report from her surgery. The report came back as decidedly Her2 negative!

When Charity's encapsulated tumor was surgically removed, the biopsy came back with no Her2 positive cancer, but it did reveal another type of cancer. Because the doctors did not want to leave any stone unturned, they decided to treat Charity with chemotherapeutic drugs for both types of breast cancer. Charity asked me for a Healing when she was feeling very ill from the chemotherapeutic drugs.

I performed another Healing for Charity.

She reported feeling rejuvenated and was able to finally get out of bed.

(I remember her telling me she started unpacking boxes immediately after her Healing.)

Then Charity started to develop neuropathy in

her feet from a new chemotherapeutic treatment that she had just started. So, I suggested that we have another Healing Session, which we did.

After her Healing, the neuropathy was completely gone!

(I am so happy for her. She is doing really well and as of this writing is two years cancer free! She is one strong warrior!!!)

MY LOYAL FRIEND

"My intercessor is my friend as my eyes pour out tears to God." (Job 16:20)

This testimony is from my loyal soul friend, who was always there for me in my darkest hours.

"I had major surgery removing infected, eroding mesh from my abdominal area. After surgery, problems persisted; infections, (including MRSA), bleeding and a perforated bladder.

"I turned to Bev for help using her healing energy abilities even though we lived at different locations. My sessions involved lying in bed alone; clearing my mind, only concentrating on my abdominal health issues. I began to feel anxiety reductions; tingling sensations where I had placed my hands on troubling abdominal areas and eventually fell into a peaceful sleep.

"Shortly after my healing session Bev phoned and was spot-on with her diagnosis of problem areas even before I was told exactly what was happening to my body.

"I had several additional sessions with comparable

results feeling better/stronger after each healing.

"I feel that energy healing triggers your immune system, promoting health and healing of body and mind. Today I am doing well, very grateful for Bev's help and highly recommend energy healing."

(I could feel the hole in my friend's bladder and could feel The Energy smoothly sealing it over. I was doing Healing Sessions on her every other day. My loyal friend was in serious trouble with massive infection throughout her abdomen and a hole in her bladder, but because of her Faith in God and trust in what I do, she came through with flying colors!)

. . . And she lived!!!

HER LONG-STANDING FORTITUDE

"To each of us is given the manifestation of the Spirit for the common good. For to one is given through the Spirit . . . the gifts of healing." (1 Corinthians 12:7-10, 29-30)

This next client had been plagued by persistent tinnitus in her ears. Her family scheduled a Distance Healing and the client reported a 50% reduction in the tinnitus after the Healing.

This client had also been suffering from rheumatoid arthritis for decades that was getting progressively worse. She could no longer stand at work and needed aids to be able to walk.

Her family member had contacted me to schedule a Distance Healing. The next morning after the Healing, my client got up automatically and walked normally from her bed to the bathroom without the use of her walking aids! We were all very joyful and awestruck!

. . . and she walked!!!

A few months later, my client's family contacted

me again for a Healing on her knee. One of her knee caps had moved down on her leg and had to be repositioned. She also was harboring staphylococcus bacteria from a previous knee surgery. Again, I felt the seriousness of the situation and suggested a Prayer Healing for the family to participate in. The client felt tingling behind her knee cap and felt the knee cap being moved during the Healing. The family members who prayed also felt tingling, electricity-like sensations during the Healing.

The Amazing thing about this Healing was that my client had actually felt her knee cap being moved without any physical manipulation being done on it!!! It was being Healed energetically, over a great distance.

God's Healing Energy was also felt by the family members who Prayed for my client during her Healing.

I am always amazed at how laser focused these Distance Healings have been. The Divine Energy that is sent to Heal my clients does what is needed at that particular time on this earth for the highest and greatest good of my clients.

Faith, direct intention, openness, connection and Prayers are all essential components that invite The Divine to perform these Miraculous Healings. God is Omnipotent and All Knowing.

He can do whatever He wishes whenever He wishes, but He wants us to be in a very personal relationship with Him.

He wants us to turn to Him in good times and in bad.

He wants us to be filled with His Holy Spirit and His Grace.

He is our Creator and loves us very much like we love our own children, only more perfectly. He loves us unconditionally!!!

A BEAUTIFUL HEART!

"Blessed are the pure of heart, for they shall see God."
(Gospel of St. Matthew 5:8)

This next client of mine was suffering from formaldehyde toxicity, which she was unknowingly exposed to in her work environment. She ended up in the ER, suffering from anaphylactic shock after using Nasonex (which contains formaldehyde as a preservative) for the first time. The doctors sent her home without connecting the Nasonex to her anaphylactic reaction.

She developed blisters all over her beautiful face. They were so bad that she was not comfortable to leave her home. Her doctors told her that her liver was toxic and that it would take at least two months to detox.

When I heard about her distress, the word Nasonex popped into my head. I then asked her if she had ever used it. She said yes, just once, right before she went into anaphylactic shock and into the ER. I offered to do a Distance Healing.

During her Healing, she started to feel tingly, electricity-like, pinprick sensations only on her blisters. She then felt a pressure on her abdomen, over her liver, which she described as if a brick was resting there. Then she started to feel like someone was pushing her up from behind her shoulders to a sitting position, which she assumed, and then she proceeded to cough and spit something out.

During her Healing, she kept seeing a Purple banner with the letters "ski" in Gold imprinted on it, running in front of her eyes. She was seeing God's Magnificent Energy then.

(I am not sure what the letters of my last name signified. Perhaps that I was being used as God's Vessel to deliver His Magnificent Healing Energy.

Gold is the color of Christ's Energy.

His Energy is one of Perfect Love, coming from His Sacred Heart.

In a vision to Saint Catherine Laboure, Mother Mary produced gold letters in the air around Herself in order to show Saint Catherine Laboure the model of the Miraculous medal that The Blessed Mother wanted her to create. I know that She walks with me, helping and Healing myself and my clients.)

My client with her beautiful heart also has a beautiful face without one scar and a totally detoxed liver!

(The Healer must also have a pure heart to send God's Healing Energy. One must never do a Healing while less than loving and positive.)

FORGIVENESS

". . . and forgive us our trespasses as we forgive those who trespass against us." (Based on Matthew 6 :12)

This next Healing was a very Mystical Healing.

My client stated that she was lying in a relaxed state, listening to meditation music, for about 45 minutes during her Healing session. After she arose, she reported feeling a burning sensation begin in the area around a surgical site.

During her Healing session, she had asked that forgiveness and compassion fill the space of her surgical site. She stated that she was having anger issues with people who had behaved badly, and she wanted to replace any angry and hateful feelings towards them with compassion and forgiveness instead.

She described the burning feeling as laser like. She stated that this feeling was uncomfortable, but that it was not agonizing.

As she awoke the next morning, she said she began to visualize a cream-colored satin case with a green velvet outline that was positioned in the surgical space

She reported seeing a ruby, in the shape of a diamond, which she believed was the stone that signified the love that she needed.

She also reported seeing a round amber stone next to the ruby, which she believed signified compassion.

She also reported seeing a diamond in the shape of a snowflake, which she believed to signify each unique circumstance that she needed to forgive.

She stated that in the middle of these three stones that were arranged in a triangular configuration, with the diamond being the apex at the bottom, was a soft blue sapphire that radiated peace.

She stated that she felt that she was being mined, so to speak, to find these stones and that she felt that their results were her intention that she had set for her Healing to herself.

(Before I begin a Healing, I always ask my clients to set their intentions clearly and specifically for what they would like to receive from the Healing.)

Most times my clients' Healings happen immediately as I am performing their Healings on them. Sometimes they happen a little later on in time as this one did and very rarely, they have occurred before my actual physical performance of the Healing. A few Master Reiki Healers have been able to do this. I feel so incredibly Blessed to have been anointed with this Amazing Gift!

ETERNAL LIFE

"So, we fix our eyes not on what is seen, but on what is unseen, since what is seen is temporary, but what is unseen is eternal." (2 Corinthians 4:18)

This Healing was an even more unique and unusual circumstance than normal for me.

It was unique because this was the first Healing that was sent to a wonderful soul who had already left her physical body. She was a wife and mother who was fighting very hard to stay here on this earth; fighting very hard not to leave behind her beloved husband, children, grandchild, family and friends.

She was in a coma and when she finally died; her body was taken away in order to harvest her organs. After quite some time had passed, nurses came out to inform the family that she had a heartbeat and started to breathe on her own again!

She tried very hard to speak and would respond to people who would pray or speak to her by turning her head towards them.

In the end, unfortunately, she did not win her

fight to stay here on this earth and it became time for her to pass.

During the afternoon of her passing, shortly before she passed, I kept hearing a voice in my head that repeatedly kept saying her name, over and over again.

I felt agitated and very strongly compelled to call her friend to see how she was doing and to offer my help if needed.

Her friend contacted the family about my experience and found out that this strong fighter had passed. She passed about an hour after I had called her friend to ask if I could help.

Her friend then contacted me during dinner with the very sad news.

I was obviously very upset and disappointed. I had hoped that maybe a Healing could have kept her here on Earth with her loved ones. I tried to eat my dinner, but I couldn't even taste it.

In spite of the devastating news of her passing, I still felt that I was needed. I told my husband how I was feeling, and he suggested that I perform a Healing even though this beautiful soul had already left her earthly body. So, I called my friend again and told her how I felt and offered to do a Healing an hour later after I finished my dinner.

Before I started the Healing, I asked God, Jesus, and the Angels to guide me as I was walking into unchartered territory. I had never performed a

Healing before on a soul that had already left its earthly body.

Almost immediately after I started the Healing, I saw a bright deep Violet/Purplish light that was framing a bright White Light inside. My intuition told me to ask that this soul be guided to the Light and to pass safely through the portal that I had seen behind my eyes. I repeatedly asked for this during the Healing. At the end of this Healing, I felt a profound sense of peace and calm. I knew that she was safely escorted Home to God and Jesus by the Angels.

She truly lives now in Heavenly Peace.

(This beautiful Violet/Purple Light frame that surrounded the White Light was also seen by her minister. Her minister saw it hovering over the girl who had just passed, while she lay in her hospital bed.

In addition, this same minister saw this same beautiful Violet/Purple frame that surrounded a brilliant White Light, at the funeral. She saw this beautiful departed soul come through this framed portal of Light. She appeared more translucent than her earthly body and she glided weightlessly over to her loved ones to bounce above their heads.

She was smiling radiantly with joy!

Her minister was sensing that she was trying to tell her grieving family that there was no more sadness, fear, pain or regrets, only deep, unconditional love for all of them. She and her sister, who also had passed, no longer wanted them to be sad, grieving or hurting in any way over their passing.

She seemed to be tethered to the Light and then she turned around to face her sister who had also passed and who was waiting for her inside the portal with an outstretched hand. She reached in through the portal and took her sister's hand.

While glancing back at her loved ones she went smiling radiantly back through the portal into the Light! Then the portal suddenly closed.

I have no doubt that she is in a Magnificent Place!)

Many neuroscientists try to explain their patients' near-death experiences, where the patients often describe seeing a very bright White Light, often finding themselves traveling towards this Light in and through a tunnel, as a pre-wired function of our human brains. They claim that humans are wired to experience this during the death of our bodies.

Well I am here to tell you that I and this lovely girl's minister certainly did not die nor did we have a near death experience!

We are alive and well to tell you that we both had the same vision, we both were a very great distance from each other and we both do God's work. I'll let you decide. . . .

THE BREATH OF LIFE

"Then the Lord God...breathed into his nostrils the breath of life." (Genesis 2:7)

This next Healing was sent remotely to a very good friend of mine. Here is his description of his Healing.

"Twenty-eight years after I quit smoking, my annual physical resulted in a diagnosis of IPF-idiopathic pulmonary fibrosis, or emphysema, or asthma, or asthma or. . . . Whatever, I could not breathe. The measured breathing test showed 35% of normal breathing capacity and a great need for some miracles. My internist told me to lose a lot of weight. I did.

"Prayers at the Mission San Juan Capistrano with Frere Junipero Serra (now Saint Serra) brought my breathing back to 53% of normal. Both the medical profession and the God profession says minimally a near miracle.

"Then a 5% reversion. My friend Bev, a recognized energy healer, said let's give it a try. We picked a time. I was at home on the bed with soothing music turned on and my eyes closed. I did not go to sleep. I was not awake. Ethereal floating. Suspended thoughts in the clouds. Gentle magnetic waves of energy drifting around me, above me, through me. A clean clear mind.

"After about an hour, I awoke in serenity. Not like a near-death experience – have experienced more than one – not like passing to eternity or visiting the pearly gates, but white and gold.

"Peace. Love.

". . . At the next breathing test, I regained the lost ground."

(Another interesting thing about this Healing was that my friend got up at the exact moment I finished his Healing, even though I told him not to move for at least an hour. He knew exactly when it had ended.)

My dear friend needs to have surgery soon and his doctor advised him to try to improve his breathing capacity even more, so he asked me for another Healing. During this Healing, he reported feeling a sensation like warm rain. He also fell asleep during the Healing. A few days after his Healing, he texted me saying that he was breathing a lot smoother.

My dear friend was scheduled to see his surgeon to have a consultation regarding the best and safest way to perform a potentially dangerous surgery for a problem that his doctors now felt needed to be addressed.

I offered to do another Healing for him before he went to his big appointment.

During this Healing, my friend felt like he was actually transcending his body. He reported feeling as if all the Energy of the Universe was coming to a focal point and targeting directly on him.

At his appointment at a major medical center and teaching hospital, the doctors actually changed their minds about repairing his problem surgically and came up with a minimally invasive technique that vastly mitigated the risks that surgery could have posed to my friend!

Today my dear friend received even better news. The doctors concluded there was no longer a need for immediate surgery! Just a follow-up scan in 9 months!

Amazing!!!

ON THE WINGS OF LOVE
His Heavenly Healers and Messengers

"But for you who revere my name, the sun will rise with healing in its wings. And you will go out and frolic like well-fed calves." (Malachi 4:2)

It is often said that there are no coincidences. Here is the story of one of those special times of synchronicity.

I feel that I met this next client of mine through a very deliberate Divine Orchestration.

My husband and I had been planning a trip to Napa Valley for at least nine months over the coming Christmas holidays. Since my son was spending the Christmas holidays in Europe with his then girlfriend and her family, we were very much looking forward to traveling, so we wouldn't feel so sad about not being able to spend Christmas with him.

The whole nine months, I kept hearing a message in my head that kept repeating "don't go to Napa."

The closer the time came to our trip, the more insistent the message became. So, I thought, "well we can stay in Sonoma." That did not work out because I found out they had a cat and I am allergic to cats. I cancelled them and re-reserved my original reservation back in Napa. Well, that did not work out either because they started accepting dogs in our favorite cabin. Yes, allergic to dogs also. We were bound and determined to go away over Christmas, so we decided on a beautiful ocean town that we could drive to fairly easily. After a four-hour drive in torrential rains, we checked into a very beautiful historic hotel.

On Christmas Eve, we decided to go into town for the afternoon to do a little local wine tasting and stay for Christmas Eve dinner. I met my client that fateful afternoon.

As we were enjoying our wine, we overheard two people speaking about their studies in Energy Healing. My husband told them that I was a Reiki Healer.

They were very interested in hearing about the results of some of my Healings. We had a very pleasant time together. I offered to perform a Distance Healing Session for one of our new friends when I got home so that she could experience what it was like to receive Reiki.

A few weeks later, she contacted me and asked if my offer was still good. I said, "Of course it was!"

Here is her very eloquent description of her Beautiful Healing.

"Yesterday I had the wonderful opportunity to set up a healing with Bev. I have been struggling all year with a myriad of health issues caused by Leaky Gut that have ended me up in the ER multiple times in a lot of pain.

"Setup: relaxing ocean wave music playing lightly in background with the view of the ocean from my balcony. 1 candle lit surrounded by a few crystals on a little stool by my feet as I lay comfortably on a big LuvSac with my favorite crystals on my stomach and a rose quartz on my heart.

"Early on in the healing I felt tingling/bubbling on my stomach and face. I kept repeating in my head 'heal, heal, heal, you are healthy.' I briefly saw a big set of flapping wings with a golden sun background then I saw another set of wings with a sky-blue background. I knew they were not eagle wings, but wings of an angel. I was very relaxed in deep meditation. Then at about 45 minutes in my left foot out of nowhere kicked down the stool that had my crystals and the lit candle on it. Sending hot wax and crystals everywhere. I woke up flipped the candle right side up and fell back onto the LuvSac and fell right back into a deep meditation.

"This happened at the moment Beverly was working on my feet. And when she does healing work on herself, her left foot always twitches. It was my left foot that twitched and kicked down my stool. She said she saw green, blue, and purple.

Green being Archangel Raphael, blue being Archangel Michael, and purple being God. Archangel Raphael is the angel of healing and brings God's healing light to Earth. Archangel Raphael often works in tandem with Archangel Michael to clear away fear and stress, which are major factors affecting health. Although Raphael isn't named in the Bible, theologians believe he was the archangel who healed the infirm at the Bethesda pond described in the Gospels. The hospital I was born at was named Bethesda. I also had Raphael's Chrystal, Emerald, on my stomach during the healing.

"Overall this experience was very relaxing and peaceful. I feel very balanced and at peace. Thank you, Beverly Pokorski, for your wonderful healing and dedication." 😇 🖤

(Yes, my left foot does twitch during my self- healings, but God's Energy is the cause of this, as it was in this Healing.)

I also saw flashes of green and blue across the sun and violet pinkish purple around the pulsing sun that evening as I went down to the water to give thanks for this Healing.

I followed up with her again the next day and she said that she felt so amazing after her Healing that took place the day before. She went to qigong yoga class and felt that she was finally balanced internally. She had been told in the past by energy healers that her yin and yang were off, but she doesn't feel like that anymore since her Healing. Her friends also noticed and commented on her higher energy level and clarity.

A short while after her Healing, I received a text from her telling me that her stomach is finally healed and that her digestion is great! Thank you, God and His Divine Helpers for Healing this very sweet young girl!

MY GOOD SAMARITAN

"Love your neighbor as yourself." (Mark 12:31)

From the very first moment I moved to my new home near the ocean, my new neighbor has been the earth Angel sent to help, guard and guide me. I lived alone for a few months during the week while my husband stayed behind in the old house as it was being sold.

There was nothing that these Good Samaritans would not do for us. They saw us through a huge disaster of insecticide poisoning with subsequent evacuation and a myriad of smaller problems. They were always there with their unfailing help and support.

When my dear friend got sick with painful shingles, I offered to perform a Distance Healing for her, since she had just moved to a new community.

She describes her Healing Experience this way.

"I prepared for the session by lying down and relaxing to release my mind of stressful thoughts. A few minutes after the session began, I started to feel a tingling in my hands and feet that progressed to the exact site of my physical discomfort from shingles. This sensation continued throughout the session and then slowly disappeared.

"There was an immediate lessening of my shingles-induced pain and it continued to decrease until I was pain free by the next day. The pain and discomfort never returned, and I never required medication.

"Being a recipient of Bev's energy healing is an awesome experience and a way to recover from physical disorders without the side effects associated with medication.

"I am a true believer in this form of treatment."

(I thank my dear friend for her kind words, but I also thank God for sending His Divine Healing Energy to my family, friends and clients, because it is from Him that All Healing comes. I am just the vessel that He uses to conduct and transfer His Magnificent Positive Healing Energy.)

THE PRINCE OF PEACE

"Peace I leave with you, my peace I give you. I do not give to you as the world gives. Do not let your hearts be troubled and do not be afraid." (John 14:27)

The most common sensation that I, my clients and even some of their loved ones have felt during a Healing has been a profound sense of Peace, Love, calm, protection, comfort and wellbeing.

These wonderful sensations are the underlying theme that unifies all the very diverse and unique Healings, their Miracles and Divine Interventions.

(Along with this profound sense of Peace, I and many of my clients have seen and felt God's Pure White Light Healing Energy and Purple Energy.

I and two of my clients have seen and felt the vibrant Gold Energy of Christ.

I see the beautiful pink and blue lavender Energy of Mother Mary. I feel Her and Jesus guiding my Healings for myself and my clients.

I have also seen the emerald green Energy of Archangel Raphael, the blue Energy of Archangel Michael, the color Energies of the other Archangels and Angels, and the violet Energy of Saint Germaine.)

During my horrible experience with a psychophar-maceutical drug that left me with almost unbearable rebound anxiety, I found my mentor, Barbara Savin. She performed weekly Reiki Sessions on me.

These Sessions not only highly attuned me to Reiki, but they were the only thing that alleviated my horrific anxiety.

Along with feeling the magnetic, electric-like Energy entering my body from my head or Crown Chakra, I felt such a complete and utter sense of Peace and calm come over me. It was like being covered and tucked in by a fluffy down comforter of Serenity from Heaven.

It far exceeded the relaxation that I used to feel after a massage. The experience totally surrounded, penetrated and traveled through my very being. My Healer very lightly touched me. Many times, she just hovered over me with her hands.

When the Healing Sessions were finished, I never, ever wanted to leave.

I was able to get through my day without the debilitating anxiety that I was suffering from.

That was and is a truly priceless Gift!!!

Thank you, God, Jesus and Mother Mary for Your Peace. I am surrounded by It, enfolded by Love and guided by Divine Love and Light.

(I cannot honestly think of a client that did not experience this Heavenly sense of peace, calm and serenity. Actually,

many of my clients fall asleep during their Healing Sessions and some stay asleep for quite some time.)

ONE LAST GIFT

"Every good gift and every perfect gift is from above, coming down from the Father of lights with whom there is no variation or shadow due to change." (James 1:17)

This next client of mine was suffering from a very aggressive type of metastatic cancer. Her condition was very grave, and she was suffering terribly from the strong and aggressive treatments of chemotherapy that were needed to give her a chance at survival.

She was in a great deal of pain and was unable to walk. She would moan frequently from the pressure of the cancer on her brain. She understandably also suffered from anxiety.

Her faithful friend had asked me to perform a Healing on her. Her friend's daughter was going to be visiting my client, so we arranged her Healing around that visit. I actually was afraid that I was not going to be able to perform this Healing on her because during my pre-healing phone consult, my client was moaning so badly and was so agitated that I did not know how we were going to start the

Healing.

But I worked with her friend's daughter and we got her to somehow calm down and listen to the Healing music so that I could start.

After her Healing had taken place, her daughter texted me and also told her Mom that my client had a profound sense of peace and calm that they had not seen in several years, was not moaning, and they actually had a full-blown conversation! She told her Mom in utter amazement, that it was "just a Miracle!!!"

Her Mom texted me in tears of joy because after the Healing, they spoke for hours, she and my client. My client answered the phone, laughed, ate, talked without moaning, and had not referenced any pain. My client's friend texted me that it was like old times. She texted me the result of these Healings and stated that she was still walking around in total utter, amazement the next day. She stated that she felt that I was truly sent from Heaven. I feel a more accurate description of this would be that God used me to send His Gift of Heaven to them. I was so grateful that God gave these two very strongly bonded souls one last great memory of their lives together to cherish forever.

A MOTHER'S LOVE

"As one whom his mother comforts, so I will comfort you." (Isaiah 66:13)

This next Healing took place on the daughter of my client whose Healings I describe in the next chapter.

Both mother and daughter were diagnosed with breast cancer just a few months apart of each other. The mother's cancer was a recurrence and her daughter's was newly diagnosed. Needless to say, the mother was devastated. Not only did she have to navigate herself through choosing the right doctors and treatment options for herself, but now she had to worry about her young daughter who is mentally challenged. It was almost too much for their family to bear. The doctors decided to perform a double mastectomy on her daughter.

I performed a Prayer Healing the day before the daughter's surgery with her Mom participating in it, cradling her young daughter and placing her hand on her daughter's tumor because I did it via Distance Healing.

As soon as a I started the Healing, I felt a lot of

Energy surrounding me from my head down and I also felt cold. I also saw very bright Violet Purple light.

The surgery went well. All the lymph nodes were benign!

A few hours after the surgery, complications developed. Swelling and bleeding started on the right side. If they could not get it to stop, they were going to have to take her back into surgery.

My mentor, Barbara Savin, cleared her while I performed a Healing.

Within thirty minutes of starting the Healing, the daughter said that she was really hungry. Her mother laughed with relief while the nurses got her daughter applesauce.

Within an hour of starting the Healing, the swelling went down, and the bleeding completely stopped. The Healing took place for a little over an hour.

Also, the daughter never needed or took one pain medication while in the hospital for five days or at home afterwards! The nurses and surgeons were all amazed as was her Mom. Her Mom could not get her to settle down and rest when she came home because she had so much Energy after the Healing. She also suffered from a postoperative infection which required IV antibiotics that were administered at home daily by a visiting nurse and she still did not need any pain medication!

The following week, the surgeons had to go back

in and remove a large blood clot and replace an implant. My client still did not have any need for any pain medications! Truly Amazing!

(I am so grateful that God intervened to protect this pure, innocent soul!)

AN AMAZING FAITH!
An Amazing Miracle!!!

"Daughter, your faith has healed you. Go in peace and be freed from your suffering." (Mark 5:34)

This next client came to me after hearing about some of the Miracles that had happened during my Healing Sessions with my clients. My client had experienced a recurrence of breast cancer in her internal mammary lymph nodes after a nine-year remission. She was understandably very upset about the recurrence. She was frustrated because she is very religious and could not understand why this was happening to her. She was ready to give up on her praying, but her Angels told her not to quit five minutes before the Miracle. Boy am I glad she didn't! And I am quite certain that she is too!

Then she heard about my success as a distance Healer. She asked Barbara Savin for my number. When she called me, she told me that she thought that I was really curing people. Of course, when she said this to me, I proceeded to inform her that God is doing the curing, and I am just the conduit.

When I started her first Healing Session, I felt the cancer in her lymph nodes on her chest immediately as I was scanning that area. It was so pronounced that I said "whoa!" out loud during the Healing. I never speak out loud during a Healing Session. We spoke after her Healing Session and she said that she started coughing a lot about five minutes after I hung up with her from her pre-Healing phone consult. This would have been right when I started her Healing. She needed to get up and drink some water to calm the coughing down. I thought at first that it might have been her acid reflux that caused her to cough but she said that she never coughed like that before. After I hung up with her from her post-Healing consult, I started my walk on the beach to give thanks for her Healing. I immediately heard a thought in my head that suggested that maybe the cough was not caused by her acid reflux. Then I had a thought that connected her cough to the cancerous lymph nodes on her chest. I also remembered her asking me if what her Angels said about not quitting five minutes before the Miracle meant anything to me?

We did a few more Healings and I still felt the cancer, but it was feeling less and less pronounced. She would feel extremely cold during most of these Healings. During one of these Healings I opened my eyes and saw a very beautiful soft Violet Purple light hovering over her from her head down to her chest where her cancer was. I saw this Light on my Healing table.

Then she asked me for another Healing Session which we did as a prayer Healing Session. Prayers were requested for my client for the time of the entire session.

My client had a candle lit about five feet or so away from her on a night stand. During this Healing, she saw beautiful rays of Light coming from the candle directly to her chest. She also felt a prolonged burning and itching sensation on her chest where the cancerous lymph nodes were. She felt the burning sensation twice and it correlated to the approximate times that I was working on her lymph nodes. She also reported feeling very cold on her left side. I saw intense colors of Violet Purple. I also felt very intense emotion during the Healing. It felt like a mixture of strong desire to help, intention, gratitude and connection with the Divine.

I usually have tears run down my face like this during a Healing.

At the end of that very powerful Healing, I could hardly feel anything at the site of her cancerous lymph nodes. I was very encouraged to say the least, but we just had to wait and see until she could have the next CT/PET scan which wasn't to take place for two more months! All I could tell her was that it felt much, much better when she assumed that nothing had changed. I repeatedly kept telling her that she had to dig deep and keep the Faith.

When it was almost time for her to have her scan, she asked for another Healing. Again, I could hardly detect anything at the site of her cancer. She said she felt extremely cold during the Healing. At the end of the Healing, I felt a fairly large Energy bubble over her chest where her cancer was. I became concerned because I did not know what it was. Then a thought came to me that said not to worry, that it was not what I was afraid it might be, namely the cancer growing larger. As I consulted with her after this Healing, I described what I had felt and relayed what I had heard.

She also saw Barbara for a Healing after that and Barbara felt the Energy bubble also.

While we were waiting for her results from her scan, I went down to the water to pray. As I was watching the sun setting, I saw beautiful outlines of Violet Pink outlining and circling the sun. I also saw auras of bright, deep Pink and Lavender radiating outward from and surrounding the pulsing sun.

Then I saw a dark cloud come from behind the sun. It shot out small, perfectly round gray circles on either side of the sun that got progressively smaller and lighter in color. Then the thought "lymph nodes "came into my head.

And guess what? She just received the results of

her PET/CT scan today. The words on the radiology report stated, "significantly improved!!!"

She had a complete reversion to normal size and undetectable status of one cancerous lymph node and a reversion in size and to a non-hypermetabolic status of the other one!

(As I previously stated, my client still had to wait several months after her lymph node Prayer Healing until she could have her PET/CT scan.

Two weeks before her scan, she consulted with my Healer, Louisa.

My client reported to me that Louisa channeled with Jesus regarding these results and He said things were "significantly improved"!!! These were the exact same words used by the radiologist who read her scans and wrote them on the report.)

I just received an email from her today, approximately nine months after the first great PET/CT scan result that I cited in the previous paragraph. She had another follow up scan and her doctor has informed her that she is now in a full and complete remission!

She refused chemotherapy and radiation when she was diagnosed with the recurrence of her cancer. The location of these nodes makes them inoperable.

A Miracle? Me thinks so!!!

Thank you, God, Jesus, Blessed Mother Mary, Saint Jude, and all of God's Divine helpers!

MY MIRACLES AND HEALINGS

"Be still and know that I am God; I will be exalted among the nations, I will be exalted in the earth." (Psalm 46:10)

Almost ten weeks before my son's wedding, my only child, I was struck to the left side of my head by a soccer ball while coming home from my beach. I was struck from behind and had no idea it was coming. It was a pretty hard hit and it resulted in a concussion and whiplash. I was urged to visit the ER to rule out any bleeding or swelling in my brain. I really was having very mild concussive symptoms at this point. I only went for peace of mind, for myself and for those who cared about me.

After a CT scan showed a negative result for any bleeding or swelling, the attending ER physician ordered a lumbar puncture. I did not want this invasive procedure and expressed my feelings to the attending ER physician prior to the procedure. I have had some medical physician training in the past and felt his reasoning was very poor. I told him that I thought it was overkill, no pun intended! But he managed to scare the heck out of me.

My intellect and my intuition, or gut instincts as they are commonly referred to, were all screaming a big resounding NO to this procedure!

But in this case, unfortunately I did not listen to them. That turned out to be a big mistake! After consulting several highly regarded medical professionals, I later found out that this procedure had no medical merit because of the immediate negative CT test result, and the type of trauma and symptoms (and lack thereof) that I was presenting.

Of course, the results of the lumbar puncture were totally negative!

I never advocate the substitution of Reiki, the internet, your intuition or gut instincts for medical treatment.

Reiki, the internet, your intuition, and gut instincts are not a substitute for medical treatment.

Always seek the advice and care of a licensed medical/health care practitioner.

That being said, unfortunately I actually was misdiagnosed by the attending ER physician. In my case, a qualified medical second opinion was definitely warranted!

I was told I had a migraine, even though I had never had one in my life and told to go home and take magnesium!

Fortunately, my internist and my neurologist at Cedars Sinai in Los Angeles correctly diagnosed my concussion, whiplash and possible cerebral spinal fluid leak.

Immediately after the ER visit, I started experiencing constant and worsening headaches, nausea, tinnitus, neuropathy, numbness and weakness in my legs, feet and hands, especially in my left hand and foot, and general weakness and shakiness for over two months whenever I tried to stand up.

The symptoms were so severe that I could not get out of bed except for very short periods of time. I was very ill and quite debilitated.

Prior to this ER visit, I walked two miles a day up and down steep hills to the beach and never sat down during the day. After about five weeks of feeling very ill after that ER visit my mentor, Barbara Savin, suggested that I give Louisa Mastromarino, who is a holistic specialist, a call to see what she was feeling.

So, I did.

Louisa was sensing meridian misalignment in my brain caused by the force of the impact of the soccer ball.

She also was sensing a concussion, along with other physical and energetic damage, including possible nerve damage on the left side of my body and a possible problem at the site of the lumbar puncture.

Louisa also said that an Angel stepped in to save my life when the soccer ball struck my temple. As soon as she started telling me this, I felt very strong vibrations of energy traveling through and shaking my entire body.

Thank you, my dear guardian Angel, for saving my life!!!

After this very powerful Healing, where Jesus, Mother Mary, Mother Kwan Yin, many Angels and Saints were present, I was able to get out of bed the very next day!

I started to regain my strength and energy and started to feel more like my old, healthy self! I was finally feeling well enough to travel to L.A. to see my neurologist.

An MRI was ordered by my neurologist to assess the prolonged symptoms. After placing me on the MRI table, the headrest, which was not properly secured into place by the person responsible for doing so, slammed down into its proper position. This action slammed and bounced my head near the base of my skull, very hard against the back of the head rest.

This trauma resulted in severe nausea during the MRI and over a week of recurring and worsening headaches, recurring and constant nausea, and an inability to get out of bed again without weakness and shakiness for several more weeks!

Through no fault of my own, I was a mess, again.

My second Healing with Louisa took place after the MRI debacle which resulted in a second concussion.

During this very profound Healing, one of the

things that Louisa described that was happening to me was that Jesus sealed a hole in my meninges lining at the base of my skull where cerebral spinal fluid was leaking. I have no doubt that this is true because prior to that Healing, after the second hit to my head by the MRI machine head rest, I was worse than ever! I could not stand up without getting weak and shaky! Immediately after this very powerful Healing, I was able to get out of bed again with a tremendous amount of energy!

I was able to make another long trip up to Cedars Sinai hospital in L.A. to see the cerebral spinal fluid leak specialist.

And guess what? He did not think I had a cerebral spinal fluid leak!

The Doc gave me permission to make the long trip to my son's wedding! I was overjoyed and very grateful!!!

I had so much energy that I stayed in town for dinner, made the long trip back home from L.A. and stayed up well past midnight!

Before this Healing with Louisa, I was desperately ill! I had no medical intervention at this point for my symptoms because I was too ill to travel to L.A. again to see the cerebral spinal fluid leak specialist or to see a physical therapist for the whiplash. I only had Energy Healings with Louisa, Barbara and myself.

When I heard the wonderful news that there was

no leak, I was incredibly relieved and overjoyed, but the linear side of my brain still had trouble grasping the wonderful news.

I was certain that my Doc was going to tell me that I had a cerebral spinal fluid leak! I was presenting with all the symptoms of one up until the time of those two Healings with Louisa!

My Angels reminded me, as I was writing this chapter, what Louisa had told me during that Healing; namely that Jesus had sealed the leak at the base of my skull! I was so certain that the lumbar puncture was the source of the leak that my mind fixated on that without really absorbing what the Holy Spirit had revealed to me.

I heard this, but my intellect prevented me from processing it because I thought my lumbar spine was the source of the leak! Jesus was sealing the source of another leak that was most likely caused by the MRI incident. He actually is probably very amused with me right now for being such a dummy!

I must admit that I was pretty foggy and confused in my brain at that point in time, after suffering all the traumas to my head. There was also so much going on all at once in this profound Healing that I was just trying to keep up, but I still was stubbornly holding on to my intellect, instead of really hearing and absorbing what was being revealed to me without debate.

Then when I later recalled what had been revealed to me, I realized that your intellect will impede Spiritual Revelation. Openness and surrender are the qualities needed in order for us to access Divine Revelation. This was a very valuable lesson for me to learn.

It truly is about the journey and our Spiritual evolution along the way.

I felt guilty for stubbornly holding on to my erroneous intellectual assessment of the location of the leak. But I also realize that it is about forgiving ourselves when we falter and forgiving others when they do, as God always does. We all will make mistakes in life because we are living in a human body, but the important thing is that we learn from them, try not to repeat them and continue to grow closer to The Light on our Soul journey.

We need to go deep into the core of our Spiritual selves, the Sacred place where we connect with God, in order to access His Knowledge and the True Purpose for our lives.

Faith is defined in Hebrews 11:1 as "the substance of things hoped for, the evidence of things not seen."

Faith is what I bring to these Healings.

They are filled with Hope for the fulfillment of mine and my clients' intentions. I connect with our Creator in that deep, Sacred Space inside my Soul.

That is the Space where I am One with God. That

is where He resides in all of us. He is us and we are Him. He is the Source of all life, across all universes, the Eternal Light of Perfect and Unconditional Love that radiates out from our connected hearts. The evidence is undeniably there as the end results of these Miraculous Healings.

It is also evidenced by the physical sensations that I and my clients feel, see and hear during these Healings.

I cannot even begin to understand the metaphysical Powers behind all of these Miraculous Healings, but it is not important that I do. It is only important that I Believe and have Faith!

God indeed has Power over all the elements of our physical world!!!

The Spiritual supersedes the physical.

Now I know firsthand how my clients feel when God, Jesus, Mother Mary, Mother Kwan Yin, the Angels, Saints, Spirit Guides and other Ascended Masters facilitate Miracles for them!

(After my son's wedding, I went back to Cedars to have a special 3D MRI myelogram done and it confirmed that there was no cerebral spinal fluid leak!

This negative diagnosis corresponded directly with the disappearance of my symptoms after my Healings with Louisa! The first Healing sealed the hole left by the lumbar puncture and the second Healing sealed the hole in the base of my skull that must have been caused by the blow to my head by the MRI headrest.)

I made it to the town where my son was getting married. It took us two days to drive there because of the bumps on the roads that did aggravate my concussions and whiplash.

After our first dinner with my son and his fiancé, I suffered a very minor jostle to my body when the elevator landed at the bottom floor of our bed and breakfast hotel. No one else even noticed this landing, but because I had suffered two concussions by then, the nausea, headaches and symptoms returned with a vengeance. I was in bed again, Praying that I would not miss the rehearsal dinner and my son's wedding. I was already missing a small wine and cheese reception. The next morning, I was not feeling much better. The rehearsal dinner was that evening!

My husband suggested that I call Louisa. That was among the best advice he has ever given me. Louisa performed another Healing and I was able to get out of bed with increasing energy and disappearance of symptoms. I was able to attend the rehearsal dinner, the beautiful wedding that took place the next day and the going away brunch the following day! Each day my stamina and energy increased while my symptoms dramatically disappeared!!!

During each of my Healing Sessions with Louisa, I could feel a tremendous amount of Energy encircling me and flowing through me. I felt strong magnetic-electrical sensations of tingling currents and waves of Energy during these psychic, energetic Healings. After each of my Healings with Louisa, I was able to get up out of bed and felt stronger and more energetic. My prior symptoms would disappear.

I felt like my old self!!!

Louisa said that I had more people Praying for me than anybody has ever had before. I requested Prayers from my spiritual friends. Several other wonderful people added me to their Prayer lists and Prayed individually for me.

I thank all of those kind and caring Souls who Prayed for me!

I thank them all for their Love and support.

Prayers absolutely realize Miracles!!!

When I look back on how sick I was before those Miraculous Healings, I know that there was no way I could have been well enough to attend my son's wedding! I could hardly even get out of bed! I desperately wanted to be there to see my son get married. I was in desperate need of a Miracle!

I got Them! Big time!!!

I thank You God, Jesus, Mother Mary, Mother Kwan Yin, Archangels Michael, Raphael, and Melchizedek, Saints Jude, Augustine, Padre Pio, Father Serra, and all of God's Angels, Saints and Divine Healers who were there for me and who performed these Magnificent Miracles!!!

(Louisa had just told me recently that the Angels

applauded me because they didn't know how I got to that wedding.

Well, I know. . . . It was by God's Good Grace and His Divine Healers, Jesus, Mother Mary, Mother Kwan, other Ascended Masters, the Angels and the Saints that I was able to attend!)

MY MARIAN HEALING

"From now on all generations will call me blessed, for the Mighty One has done great things for me . . . holy is his name." (Luke 1:46-55)

From the very start of my Amazing Journey, the Blessed Mother Mary has always been with me.

She has walked beside me on the shore at the water.

(As I mentioned before, two light workers have told me this. One of them was a complete stranger to me at the time.)

She was with us after my dear Mother's funeral.

She has walked beside me in my home as witnessed by her beautiful pink Energy coloring my white floor tiles.

She has been with me in my car and where I park to go down to the water.

The whole sky would turn bright pink when it would be time for me to go down to the water and take my videos. No one else could see her beautiful Energy. Believe me, I asked several people!!!

She has moved the sun and the moon in visions and on video. I have captured her shadow on a picture taken by my cell phone in the beach parking lot after I returned from giving thanks for my client's Miraculous Healings.

(I would always go down to the water to give thanks after a Healing and to capture my pictures and videos of the sun.)

She helps me fight the good fight!!!

A few months before my first concussion and whiplash occurred, we were sitting on a plane in New York, waiting to take off for Rome.

I am quite terrified to fly, so this was quite a feat for me. We had just arrived in New York after flying cross country from LA. We were supposed to meet our son in New York and head on out to Rome together. But as luck would have it, weather delayed his flight in and he got to the gate just as they had closed the doors. I was so upset. There was no way that he was getting on that plane and there was no way they were going to let me get off.

Then the pilot came on the speaker to inform us that we would be flying into some pretty rough storms over the Atlantic. Well, as anyone who is nervous about flying in great weather knows, you can imagine the panic that I was experiencing.

I started Praying while holding onto my cross bracelet, like my life literally depended on it. About ten minutes or so later, the pilot came on again and announced that the weather had cleared, and it would be clear sailing. And it was!

I am quite certain that my Prayers were answered by Jesus and Mother Mary.

The first site we visited in Rome was the Vatican. I could not wait to see Michelangelo's Pieta, the sculpture of the Virgin Mary holding her deceased Son.

The videos that I took of this incredibly beautiful work of art, were actually shaking. In one, the whole video was vibrating and in others the sun light coming through the small windows was flashing.

We ended our stay in Italy in Positano.

Not only was it the most stunning coastal town I had ever seen but I felt so much peace there.

I was so grateful that I was able to experience that beautiful country with all its spiritual history because a few months later my injuries began.

Shortly after I was Healed from the whiplashes and concussions, I developed a bladder problem. I was given an antibiotic called Levaquin by a gyne-cologist.

After only two doses, I suffered severe, adverse side effects and had to stop the medication. It caused severe tremors and palpitations in my chest. I had quivering down my legs from my waist down. It felt like a nuclear bomb had gone off in my body!

I then developed tendinitis and pain all over my whole body, especially in both my ankles, knees, hamstrings and hands. My joints would pop, and my muscles and bones would hurt. I had constant neuropathy and pain that did not allow me to sleep.

I developed PTSD and word recall problems.

My skin would burn and started to peel off. These were the most offensive of the side effects I had experienced.

There were other less severe ones also.

I was unable to walk down my stairs for months, drive for almost five months or even put my feet up to rest on my heels. I had to use a wheelchair to walk anywhere but short distances.

As one can imagine, I struggled to stay positive. Tendons take a very long time to heal because of their poor vascularization and innervation.

I tried to stay positive and do Reiki on myself, but I was in a great deal of pain all over my body and was just too tired. I was completely debilitated. I could no longer perform Healings for my clients or go down to the water where I would find my peace and Healing.

Then came my lowest day ever!

I was enveloped by a deep despair.

I just did not think that I could endure any of it anymore. That's when Divine help came!!!

My iPad was charging on the kitchen counter. The screen was completely black. No tabs were open.

My husband brought it into the bedroom and what I saw on that previously black screen helped me to face another day! It was a live recording of my new grandbaby on the Baby cam.

I have no idea how that could have happened! And as my husband left the bedroom, a ceiling fan in the living room that cannot be turned on, except with a remote that is always in a cabinet, was spinning full blast! We NEVER turn on any of our ceiling fans because of my allergies.

I watched that video tape of God's precious Gift to me for three days straight! The despair did not return. Again, I was rescued by The Divine!!! I am so very grateful!!!

I started working with Louisa again to try to accelerate my Healing.

I was guided to a fantastic physical therapist. I started making slow but steady progress when I could finally get down the stairs to start therapy.

Then Mother Mary decided to take over my Healing on my legs and ankles. (She had already Healed my bladder by then.)

After each Healing Session with Louisa, I would fall into a deep sleep in the middle of the afternoon. I never take naps during the day because I wake up feeling very groggy and then have trouble sleeping at night. But this deep sleep would overtake me beyond my control.

I started to have more mobility with less pain and

swelling after each Healing.

My mood would improve. I started to feel hope again! I never gave up!!!

After a few Healings like this, along with instructions to resume my self-Healings, I felt the desire to edit my book again.

As soon as I sat down and opened my computer to reveal my manuscript, I felt an extremely strong Energy surround my whole head, the right side of my face and my right shoulder. It was tingling and electrifying so strongly, with an intensity like I never felt before! It stopped for a few minutes when my husband came in to move my chair for me. When he left, I resumed editing my book and mentally wondered if whoever had been there would come back. Immediately, She did!

The strong tingling started again at the top of my crown and then it went into both of my legs from my waist down to my feet. My legs were seriously vibrating on the inside!!! It felt as if something was entering them, filling them and moving down to my feet.

I thought it was Mother Mary because shortly after, I could not stay awake any longer and had to lie down in bed. This was the middle of the afternoon again. I was out cold for hours!

(This extreme sleepiness has happened for two days in a row also after a Healing with Mother Mary.)

The very next morning, I called Louisa for another Healing Session and told her what happened the day before. She confirmed what I thought; that the Energy I felt was Mother Mary.

She came to Bless my book and to Heal my legs so that I could start Healing others again, drive again and run with my grandbaby soon! So, we had a Session that morning and that afternoon I was actually able to drive my car for the first time in almost five months!

I was ecstatic!!! I am starting out slow to be safe per my doctor's instructions. I also walked down a long path to look at the ocean without using my wheelchair!

It was like Mother Mary somehow inhabited my legs and ankles with Her own. I don't know how, but I know that I felt Her do it and I witnessed the Amazing results!!!

That evening after that tremendous Marian Healing, I awoke in the middle of the night with a serene and energizing feeling that lasted for over two hours. I then drifted back off into a peaceful sleep.

I felt very peaceful and content. Mother Mary often comes in the middle of the night after a Session with Louisa. I believe that is what I felt. I usually awaken during or right after She or the Angels come.

After these sessions, I had yet another Healing Session with Mother Mary and Louisa. I then went to my physical therapy appointment the following morning.

My therapist decided to measure my ankle degrees of motion. They both went from a minus twenty degrees to zero degrees. A plus twenty degrees is normal.

That meant that I had made a fifty percent improvement, literally overnight!

I recently graduated into my walking sneakers after not being able to get into them for seven months. I went to my favorite cliff at the water that faces my Healing cliff. The sun was starting to set, but it was shining very brightly on me. A thought came into my head to shoot a video on my cell camera.

So, I immediately did.

I shot an incredible video of the sun flashing and lighting up the whole sky! A short while later after that Amazing Healing and video, I was able to walk up a slight slope that I had not been able to do easily since my injuries to my tendons.

A very interesting event occurred that same morning. I was sitting in my Healing room, looking out at the ocean when I heard loud banging noises coming from my fireplace. At first, I thought it was a golf ball, but then it became very loud, prolonged and almost insistent. I couldn't figure out what was causing the loud poundings. As I went to the other room that faces the cross above the church, I saw a huge hawk fly off my chimney. The noises stopped and the hawk never returned.

The hawk is believed to be a messenger of Spirit. They have a higher vision and perspective as they soar on the wind and look into the sun. I believe they were calling me back on my spiritual path with laser-like focus, to finish my writings and take that video.

The very next day, I went to another very beautiful cliff to sit and watch the sunset.

Afterwards, I walked up a much longer and even steeper slope without any problem!!!

I wanted to jump for joy!!! Instead, I got all choked up with tears as I threw my hat in the air, smiled and said woo hoo!!!

And of course, I said many Prayers of thanks to Mother Mary as I am quite certain that She facilitated those Healings, along with God, Jesus and Their whole Celestial Team of Divine Healers!!!

Since these Amazing and powerful Marian Healings, I have again shot incredible videos of the sun where the whole sky would suddenly turn the brightest white and the sun would be so huge and bright that it took over the whole sky!!!

I will be sharing them with everyone on my website when this book comes out.

My Amazing Journey has had so many tremendous peaks after the lowest valleys. But I do know that God and His Amazing Grace will never give up on us. All He asks is that we Believe in Him, have Faith and Pray.

Praying does indeed realize Miracles!!!

Praising God is easy in the best of times, but when we can still do it in the worst of times, that is trust. That is Faith.

And it can indeed move mountains!!!

Thank you, Mother Mary, and of course God and Jesus from whom all Good and Great things come!!!

SELF-HEALING
My Devotion

"I thank Christ Jesus our Lord, who has strengthened me, that He considered me faithful and appointed me to service." (1 Timothy 1:12)

Most days I perform Healing on myself. My intentions are to become closer and more attuned to God's Energy, and to receive physical, mental, emotional, and Spiritual Healing. I am able to find courage, strength, compassion, tolerance, peace and forgiveness. It is a Great Source of comfort and strength for me. During my self-Healings, I dedicate these positive intentions to God and pray that His Holy Spirit will continue to Bless me with the ability to receive and transfer His Love and Healing.

Here is an example of one of my most recent self-Healings.

Along with the concussive traumas to my head, I also suffered from whiplash. When I got back from my son's wedding, I realized that I didn't really even notice this before because I tried not to move my head in order to avoid the resulting pain and headaches that any movement caused from the concussions and lumbar puncture. My neurologist ordered physical therapy for the whiplash near the beginning of this trauma, but I could not get out of bed for over eight weeks to even get to a therapist!

So, when I got home from the wedding, I felt that I was well enough to try to find a therapist nearby so that the bumps in the roads would not aggravate my headaches. I was having trouble finding one. At one point, I was constantly getting disconnected while speaking to one about his experience, while trying to schedule an appointment! Hmmm....

It was then that I decided to perform a self-Healing, where I included the Healing of the whiplash as my intention and placed my hands on my neck, along with the other areas that needed Healing.

After two sessions of Healing, I was able to move my head and neck from side to side with almost full and complete range of motion restored. I started driving again after the second session!

I am so grateful for the freedom this Healing gave me! It has given me a very important part of my life back again!!!

I have also had to learn the value of balance and rest in my life. I have had to learn to slow down and take care of myself also so that I could more effectively take care of others.

Here is another example of one of my self-Healings.

My husband and I met my son and his then girlfriend in Utah to spend the Thanksgiving holiday together. We stayed high up on the mountain in Snow Bird. This was my first visit to this altitude of about 11,000 feet at the summit.

The very next morning I woke up with altitude or mountain sickness. I had no idea what was wrong. I was feeling pretty awful! My son, who had been there many times, of course knew what it was.

We had a big Thanksgiving feast coming up that afternoon and I was so nauseous that I knew there was no way I would be able to enjoy it, let alone eat it!

So, as our room had a wall of floor to ceiling windows that was directly on and facing the mountain, I asked everyone to leave me alone for a while so that I could Heal myself of the altitude sickness. I desperately wanted those Thanksgiving goodies, especially the pumpkin pie, as I have a big sweet tooth!

I proceeded to perform my self-Healing and after about 45 minutes, the altitude sickness left and never returned! I ate and enjoyed a huge Thanksgiving dinner that afternoon and the next day my son and I took the tram all the way up to the 11,000-foot summit!

I spent the rest of the weekend in total comfort!

This next self-Healing is very typical of what I see when I receive Reiki for myself and my clients. I usually see God's Energy behind my eyes but sometimes I see it externally, as have some of my clients.

I needed to have gum grafts on six lower teeth in a row. I was very anxious about the surgery, not only because of the pain, but because my esophagus goes into spasm when my mouth is worked on, causing me to cough. I did not want to be injured during the surgery because of the potential coughing.

I did a Healing right before going to sleep to help alleviate my anxiety. I immediately fell asleep and woke a few times but was able to go right back to sleep.

But then I woke up around dawn and started to get very worried and anxious. Stress causes the spasms to start and that they did, big time!

So, of course, I started a Healing immediately and the coughing subsided almost instantaneously! I felt very peaceful and calm for several hours before I went into surgery, even during the interminable hour wait in the surgeon's front office.

Right before the surgery began, whenever I opened my eyes, I saw this Beautiful soft Purple Light right in front of me. I did not cough once! After it was finished, I said to the surgeon that I did good and he said that I did really good!

Thank You God, Jesus, Blessed Mother Mary and

all Their Divine Helpers who were there to get me through!

ONENESS

I have been very fortunate to have been given signs from the Universe that we are all one, connected to each other by our Creator's Energy.

The first one happened when I arrived to take possession of my new home near the water. My realtor was waiting for me on the front porch with the keys to my new home.

We heard a ruckus overhead of hungry, little baby birds. We looked up to see that they were baby swallows and their mother had built two nests under the eaves over my front door. I was new to the swallows then, but my realtor told me they were good luck! Apparently, he was right because they come back every year, and every year I have had Amazing Healings in this home.

As I am finishing the final writings of this book, they have come again and built two nests this time over my double French doors on my back deck that faces my Healing table. They are truly a magnificent sight to behold when they all fly in and start swooping around their nests. They are very beautiful and graceful little birds.

When I first met one of my new gardeners, he had informed me that my gorgeous purple hydrangeas in my backyard had undergone a second blooming that season. He said that he had never seen that before with these particular hydrangeas that he had been tending for over a decade!

I told him that I was an energy Healer and that they were happy that I was moving in. We both laughed but I do believe that is what it truly meant. They have not bloomed twice in one season again, until now. As I am finishing the writing of this book about God's Magnificent Energy, they just bloomed twice again in one season, Magnificently and abundantly again!!!

I remember very vividly one of the first mornings in my new home. As I awoke and left my bedroom to look out at the ocean from my big picture window in my Healing room, I was greeted by a spectacular site. Across the whole expansive view of the water, there spanned three huge and brilliant rainbows, sitting side by side next to each other and spaced evenly apart. It was not only very brilliant and beautiful to look upon, but it also felt very peaceful and serene but with a sense of joy and celebration. This spectacular site faced and looked down upon my Healing table where most of the Healings that I write about in this book have taken place!

Shortly after I settled into my new home near the

ocean, I had a wonderful experience with three dolphins. It had been a particularly challenging day for me emotionally.

I was very distraught and upset so I decided to go down to the water to try to find some solace and much needed peace.

I was still feeling very much in despair when I suddenly noticed three dolphins riding in the curl of a wave towards me extremely close to the shore. It was truly incredible! That sight was so graceful, elegant and peaceful that it dissolved my upset and gave me the strength and courage that I needed to return with peace in my heart and conviction to solve my problems.

This outcome is not surprising to me since dolphins are associated with peace, harmony and inner strength.

Shortly after that, we were evacuated from our new home because of insecticide poisoning. It was a terrible experience, but our insurance took great care in housing us immediately in a wonderful hotel. Actually, there was no clause in our insurance policy that covered the incident. So naturally, I prayed very hard for a solution because we could not afford the very expensive clean up. The very next day the insurance company approved our request. Our insurance adjuster said that he had never see anything like this before! Thank God!!! I know that He had orchestrated it.

It was a very stressful time because our health was also compromised, and we were not even sure if we would be able to have a successful cleanup. It was a huge disaster.

One day when I was walking along the beach below the hotel where we were living during the cleanup, a couple came up to me and asked me to take a picture of a tribute they had made on the sand to their deceased nephew. I tried to comfort them and told them about my situation. We all held hands in Prayer for each other. Perfect strangers coming together to help each other. It was a perfect moment of unconditional love. After they left, I walked back along the beach and saw one solitary, very small whale jumping out of the water and doing multiple flips as it swam in front of me. What a wonderful afternoon it was!

The whale is associated with emotional and physical healing. Whales also value connection to one another in community.

A few Mother's Days later, I was missing my son tremendously. He lived across the country and we hadn't spent Mother's Day together since he had moved.

I was sitting on the beach, looking down at my cell phone and talking to him when something urged me to look up.

Directly in front of me, almost on the shore, was a huge humpback whale that surfaced and blew water out of its spout then proceeded to go back out to sea and swim away. Everyone around me thought it was a beached whale at first because it was that close!

That whole afternoon a small family of whales came to play in the water on the beach right in front of us. A very rare occurrence for both of these experiences.

These particular whale experiences occurred right before I became inspired to write this book. The whale signifies rebirth and, in my case, I think it was encouraging me to give birth to this creation, this book which describes the Miracles that God had created during my Healing Sessions.

As I am writing about these wonderful whale experiences, another one comes to mind. This one happened while we were vacationing in Maui over thirty years ago. My son was only four years old then and it was our first trip to the Hawaiian Islands. There was only one last family of whales left in the area. They were waiting for their baby to get big enough before they could move on.

We saw them right next to our whale watch boat. Just as I reached out to grab my four-year-old son, who suddenly decided to stand up on the rail of the boat in order to get a better view, the male whale did a breach and shot straight up out of the water right in front of us, right next to our boat! It did a 360-degree turn in the air.

It was a magnificent sight indeed!

(The whale is an animal that very much values the family unit.)

The night before my Prayer Healing was to take place on my breast cancer patient with the inoperable cancerous lymph nodes, an owl landed on my chimney and kept hooting quite loudly.

It would leave for a very short time but kept coming back on the roof above me wherever I was in my home. It only was there that one night . . . never before or since in all the years that I have lived there. A short while after the Prayer Healing that took place the very next day, my client had tremendous news on receipt of the results of her CT/PET scan regarding the remission of her cancer in her lymph nodes!

This visit from this very wise animal was an incredible Gift from the universe to me. The owl symbolizes power, wisdom, protection, guidance into the unknown, psychic ability and intuition.

I feel that this owl came as a sign from God and His Universe that this Prayer Healing was going to result in a Miracle! And indeed, it did!

Just as I was finishing my writings for this book, a beautiful hawk with a pinkish/yellow beak perched on my neighbor's deck that directly faces my healing table. It just sat there and stared at me for well over half an hour. It let my husband and me get very close to my large picture window to take its picture many times over. The picture window faces my Healing table and is very close to the corner of the deck where the hawk was perched.

I finally had to go downstairs to leave for an appointment and, as I started to leave my Healing room and descend the stairs, I saw it fly away and leave the deck.

The hawk is believed to be a messenger of the spirit world. I believe its message to me was to focus on finishing this book and soar to the Heavens with it, just like the hawk.

I feel very supported, protected and Blessed by God and His universe!

SPIRITUALITY, RELIGION, AND REIKI

Spirit is the very essence of our being.

It is the core of our existence. We all come from the same Source and we all share His Energy, His Spirit. God is us and we are Him.

I see religion as a structured way of teaching us these fundamental truths. All religions should be based on Love, because that is what God is.

Therefore, spirituality and religion are not and should not be mutually exclusive. My religion is God or Love. So Pure and True. It is The Eternal Light that Magnificently Shines.

I have spoken about Prayer Healings during my clients' Healing sessions.

Prayer is direct communication with The Divine. I use Prayer as a form of connection, communication, intention, intervention and request for a Healing.

This connection and communication can also come from The Divine to us in the form of Inspiration and Guidance from a variety of sources.

They can come as thoughts, messages, dreams, signs, written and verbal teachings, a sense of Knowing and

Inspirations.

I think it is very important to discuss the difference between doing a formal Reiki Healing on a person and Praying for a person to Heal, whether it be physically, mentally, emotionally, psychologically or spiritually.

As I previously mentioned, a person's Soul or Energy Essence is the very core of their existence. It is Sacred, originating from The Creator.

It is not ethical to send another Soul a Reiki Healing without their permission.

This is a violation of their energy, personal privacy and Reiki ethics. We are given the Gift of free will by our Creator and that means that we have the right to choose whether we want to receive a Reiki Healing or not. This decision is ours and only ours and it must be respected.

However, it is permissible to do a Reiki Healing without permission only when the person is an infant or a very young critically ill child or is in a coma or is literally in a life and death situation. In all of these situations, the person is unable to speak for themselves. Even when facing these very grave situations, I have then asked a close loved one or family member for permission to do the Healing, along with the person's own Soul and Spirit Guides.

That being said, it is permissible, desirable and wonderful to Pray for another person to receive Healing through Divine Intervention.

God, Jesus, Mother Mary, the Archangels, Saints and Ascended Masters will intervene and work with the person's own Angels and Spirit Guides in order to help them if they so choose.

But the Soul has to want the Healing and the Soul has to accept the Miracle!

The Divine Beings that have come to my personal Healings and to my clients' Healings exist in a Realm that is of God. They love us, want what is best for us and come to guide and help us. Mine has truly been an Amazing Journey with The Divine!

I, my loved ones, and my clients have been Magnificently Blessed!

VALUABLE LESSONS

As I travel along this Amazing Journey with the Divine, I continue to learn valuable lessons along the way.

When I first entered on my Amazing Journey, it would probably be fair to say that I had Faith the size of a mustard seed. That tiny seed was there, but it lay dormant because I really was very preoccupied with my earthly life of raising a family and just being a good mom and daughter to my own dear son and Mother. I was involved with helping my family, friends and neighbors. Outside of the psychic experiences that were starting to occur, I really did not become Spiritually awake until after my beloved Mother had passed. She was my very best friend and confidante. Finding out about the afterlife and Spirit world was my way of staying close to her and keeping her with me. I knew in my heart that her Mother's love for us was still very much alive and that her Spirit was all around us, watching over and helping us.

She has shown me that she is very much alive and well, living joyfully in the afterlife or Heaven!

I was very open to receiving Reiki from my very first session. That openness to God's Energy grew from Faith the size of a tiny grain of mustard seed, that was ignited, inflamed and enlarged, to the Miracles that have happened for myself and my clients.

Jesus said that you only need to have faith the size of a tiny mustard seed in order to move mountains. He said nothing will be impossible for you.

And certainly nothing is impossible for God!!!

I have learned to trust in God because He is an Awesome God!!!

I have learned to let go, surrender to God and go with the flow.

I have learned that my intellect, while it serves me well, will impede in receiving Revelation from The Holy Spirit.

I have learned that this is a Gift given to me by God that is to be protected and cherished and that its Power has nothing to do with me other than my showing up with Faith and asking with Pure and direct intentions.

I have learned that a person's Soul must accept the Miracle. God gives us the Gift of free will. This determines whether we will choose to believe and be open, or closed, to the Gift of God's Miracles. Even avowed atheists have been converted after witnessing The Divine in action!!!

I have learned what it truly means to serve:

selfless, without conditions or credits. It really is all about our service to our fellow human beings and how we go about following our calling and true Soul purpose here on this earth.

I have learned not to expect gratitude but to always express it to God for the Greatness that He is and all that He does, in a Healing and in my life.

I have learned to leave my ego behind and replace it with humility. God's Magnificence outshines anything I have ever seen or known!!!

During my traumas, I learned how to receive after being in the role of giver and Healer for so long.

I have learned how to forgive. Forgiveness is essential for your own Soul and inner peace. Harboring negative feelings towards someone who has hurt you only lowers your energetic vibration and drains your energy. It is so much better to choose to vibrate higher and shine positive Light into the world and Universe.

I find it very helpful to try to find the lesson in the middle of a painful experience and to thank the Universe for my growth because of it.

Forgiveness is an expression of love for another who has harmed you or done you wrong in some way. Physical, mental, or emotional abuse is never acceptable. But we can Pray for the souls who have hurt us.

We can view their behavior from a place of compassion and Pray for their Enlightenment and Healing.

We can Pray for Divine Intervention.

I have learned that everything happens for a reason and that it is all part of a perfect Divine plan. I may not understand it at the time that it is happening, but I have learned to trust in His infinite Wisdom because it is far Superior.

I have learned to trust and praise Him especially in difficult and trying times.

I have learned that His Deliverance will come in His Perfect timing, not in ours.

As He Himself has promised in Hebrews 13:5 that "He will never leave you nor forsake you."

And so far, He never has!!!

I have seen the tremendous power of Prayer and how it is magnified by the number of people praying. I have also learned in my own Praying experience that prayers don't always get answered in the way you would like them to. God's plan is always Superior to yours. He always provides the best solution for your Highest and Greatest Good. We often need to be still and listen for His Guidance, Direction and Divine Inspiration. This comes through the Holy Spirit who is God's extension to us on earth. It can come through Jesus, Mother Mary, Ascended Masters, our Angels, the Saints and our Spirit Guides.

Divine Guidance comes to me in many ways: through my Reiki Healing, spending time alone in nature, in the shower, (water is a great conductor of electrical energy), through dreams, through thoughts that pop into my head that are often accompanied by electrical sensations and it can also come through meditation.

I have learned to trust my intuition. This is God, Jesus, the Holy Spirit, Mother Mary, my Soul, my Angels, my Spirit Guides and my whole Divine Celestial Team of Light Beings speaking to me through thoughts and gut feelings.

It is Spiritual Wisdom.

I have seen the immediacy of the Divine in response to a need in a Healing Session. It has been mind-boggling!

Most importantly, this Amazing Journey has been about Perfect, Unconditional Love.

Because really, Love is all there is.

And our God is Love.

How Great He is!!!

CONCLUSION

As I have been approaching the end of my writings on my Amazing Journey with The Divine, I have been experiencing some very Beautiful and Miraculous visions of the sun and the moon.

They seemed to start when I began Healing Sessions on the daughter of my client, both of whom had breast cancer. I was working with them simultaneously.

I first noticed from my big picture window that faces the ocean and looks upon my Healing table, a vision of the sun at sunset that had a bright Violet Pink outline around only half of the sun, which was pulsing. The outline of Violet Pink light kept going up and down only around the left side of the sun. I kept hearing the word half. I got the impression later that these Miracles were halfway in the making.

A thought then occurred to me that the daughter's cancerous tumor was on her left side. Then as I continued to do more Healings on the mother, I started seeing the sun at the water pulsing and being fully outlined in the same Violet Pink. Bright Pink and Lavender auras would appear and surround the pulsing sun. They would pulse and grow bigger and brighter. I managed to capture a picture of this, but in my picture, there appeared what looked like two suns.

One, a miniature version of what I was seeing but it was not even visible in the sky when I snapped the picture.

It pulses in my still photograph. I cannot explain this according to the physical world we live in. It can only be explained by the Power of the Divine.

This is what called me to start taking almost daily pictures of the sun.

I also captured what looks like beautiful pink balloons, red and pink tulips and pink crowns around the sun. I have also captured a figure in front of me in shadow that appears to be wearing a crown and a long robe. This shadow figure is not casting a shadow nor is it being cast from anywhere in the vicinity like all the other objects were with the sun setting behind them. I believe it is The Blessed Mother Mary.

As witnessed by the Miracles of Fatima and Medjugorje, The Blessed Mother Mary moves the sun. I since have captured more Amazing photographs and videos of the sun and the moon, pulsing, radiating, moving and looking not of this world.

Many days, in the middle of the day, the whole sky would turn bright pink. My off-white floor tiles inside my home would appear to have large pink blotches as I walked on them. They have appeared in front of me, along with God's Purple Energy, as I prepare for a healing.

I actually have captured a picture of God's Purple Energy coloring the top of my off-white tiles in my home, especially the ones under my Healing table along with Mother Mary's pink Energy.

No one else could ever see it, this beautiful Pink energy. Believe me, I asked!

But several clients and friends have seen God's White Energy and Christ's Gold Energy.

Several have seen Purple and a bright Violet energy during their Healing sessions.

I also had another vision of the moon that was very interesting because I could not capture it on my new cell phone camera, no matter how many times I tried! This is the same camera that captured all the Amazing videos and pictures of the sun.

As I was sitting alone in my Healing room one evening, a yellow light caught my attention out of the corner of my left eye. It was coming from outside my window that the cross and the church face. The church and its cross look directly down upon my Healing table.

This yellow light was a yellow moon, about one-third full at the bottom.

It was positioned slightly above the trees that sit directly beside the left side of the cross. It kept slowly but steadily moving to the right in the sky towards the cross! I ran to get my cell phone so that I could capture this second vision of the moon, but my camera was picking up everything but the vision! I even tried to capture it in the adjacent room as it kept moving to the right towards the cross and church. Eventually the moon moved past the cross and the church and disappeared below the hill that the church sits atop. It only took a very few minutes to do this. This is just not physically possible!

As I was getting very close to finishing this book, I had a third vision of the moon. It was very high in the sky and I saw it in the rectangular window above my French doors that face my Healing table. What drew my attention to it was that it was surrounded by a very bright white, veil-like aura, tinged with pink. It was moving very quickly and steadily from the top of the window frame down to the bottom of the frame.

As I was watching this phenomenon, I smelled a very beautiful, sweet scent of flowers around my head, neck and face. I could not identify the fragrance. I don't think that I ever smelled anything like it before. It only lasted for about thirty seconds or so, but it was very distinct and quite noticeable because I do not wear perfume due to a high sensitivity to smells.

This all captured my attention and interest for sure!

When the pinkish white, veiled moon was no longer visible in the rectangular window, I looked through the French doors below the window, and there it was, sitting lower in the sky but now it just looked plain yellow.

As I went into the adjacent room to get something, I looked at it again from the other set of French doors there and it was sitting even lower in the sky now.

Less than a minute had passed by the time I saw it in the adjacent room. I was quite curious to see if anything else was going to occur. After watching and waiting for about a minute or two, I was about to leave when I heard a voice in my head that kept urging me to wait.

So, I did.

All of a sudden, the yellow moon started steadily descending towards and then went below the trees that sit to the left of the cross and the church.

Then it completely disappeared. I looked at my kitchen clock. This all took place in less than a minute!

The Blessed Mother moves the sun, as witnessed by thousands at the Miracles of Fatima and Medjugorje. I believe that She was also responsible for the three visions of the moon that I experienced. She is the Queen of Angels and is often portrayed with the crescent moon beneath Her feet. The moon reflects the light of the sun, and in these portrayals, it signifies the Light of Christ being reflected onto the moon.

All three of these moon visions took place around the cross that is the symbol of Christ.

Our Blessed Mother Mary wants to show the world that God and His Son exist, Her beloved Christ child also.

She loves us and the world, and She wants people to benefit from Energy Healing. I have been told that these Amazing visions have been shown to me because I am a visionary in using distance Energy Healing.

Since these beautiful visions of the sun and the moon that I have seen, I have had two additional visits of a brilliant white and gold being of light and a bright gold being of light.

The first visit occurred outside of my French doors that face my Healing table and the huge Cross behind it.

My home was completely dark as I was on my way to bed. I noticed two blinding flashes of white light coming kitty corner around the left side of the French doors that face my Healing table. It got my attention! I stayed to see what they were and then a beautiful being of brilliant white light appeared in front of the left French door. The being had a gold light radiating from its center. The being was approximately two feet wide and three feet tall and resembled a star.

I do not know how long it stayed there because

eventually I went into my bedroom to get ready for bed.

I do know that gold signifies Christ Consciousness.

The second visit occurred a few weeks later, outside of a small window that sits over my bed. As I was getting ready for bed again, a beautiful bright gold light being, resembling the shape of the previous star-like being that appeared outside my French doors, was hovering in the sky right outside my window, up close and personal. I stared at it for a while, then turned to put on my pajamas. It was still there when I turned back around to look at it, but it started to look a bit dimmer, so I decided to grab my cell phone and take a picture.

By the time I turned around to snap a picture, it was gone.

I also see and feel my Angel guides daily through flashes of colors, especially violet, blue, green and pale purple light, coming from the corner of my eyes. I get their validations of important messages through tingling, electrical sensations and waves of Energy around and through my body. This is the way they communicate with me as I am being guided or inspired by thoughts that pop into my head or their way of validating something important that was told to me or that I needed to know. That is how I know the guidance was from them and that they are always with me, guiding, assisting, and protecting me.

Our guardian Angels also like to make their presence known by leaving coins for us to see. One day as I was coming back to my car after my walk on the beach, I noticed a handful of coins on the ground in front of my trunk in the shape of a J. They also like to leave feathers in unusual places. One day as I was walking along the beach, looking for a ledge to sit on and absorb the wonderful peace and positive energy of the ocean, I laid my towel down on the perfect spot of sand. There was only sand, nothing else. A little while later, as I was getting up to leave, I gently picked up my towel to fold it, and underneath it was a white feather, sitting straight up in the air out of the sand! Not possible because I was just sitting on that spot of sand for quite a long time. It would have been flattened by the weight of my body, plus it was not there when I gently placed the towel down to sit on the ledge.

When I finally set the wheels in motion to start publishing my book, I sat down next to my Healing table to reflect and give thanks to God, Jesus, Mother Mary and the Angels for all of the guidance and direction that I had received.

As soon as I sat down, I felt the sun break through the clouds and shine on my face through the big picture window that faces my Healing table. I smiled because I knew it was Mother Mary congratulating me. I could feel Her sweet and tender love, Her happiness and approval! As I sat there smiling with my eyes closed, I started feeling a very strong sense of joy and euphoria. It felt much like when I walked into my Mother's home after she had passed but it felt much more pronounced and prolonged. It felt as if these joyful emotions were coming from many beings, not just one. Then, behind my eyes I started to see Violet/Purple, but it was coming in strong pulsing waves of circular lights. As I was wondering what was happening, I received a thought that said it was my Angels dancing!

I smiled and then it started to get very strong. I became a little concerned that there might still be something wrong with my vision from my concussions, so I asked that it please stop. Immediately, the pulsing and shaking stopped but the Violet Light remained.

(My Angels understood that I was feeling a bit overwhelmed at that point.)

During one of my nighttime Healings, I was allowed to see something very special. It was completely dark in my Healing room, except for some soft moonlight in the background outside. I usually don't open my eyes during a Healing session, except for very brief periods when I need to move around my Healing table. I just happened to open them and what I saw was this Pure White light bouncing off my Healing table under my hand. It was mimicking and following my hand movements very exactly and precisely as I was filling the voids for my client with God's Pure White Light Healing Energy. I kept staring at it, wondering if it was my imagination, but whenever and wherever I moved my hand, it followed and bounced.

That was just Amazing!!! God was right there with me and my distance client, validating His Presence for me.

Shortly after I had started Healing others again after I recovered from my head traumas, I had three very spectacular experiences with crosses on the same day.

I awoke that day and as I went into my kitchen to make breakfast, I happened to look at the cross that faces my Healing table. There was something different about it that morning that caught my eye and caused me to look up at it.

This normally brownish black cross was now silvery, and it was surrounded by and glowing with white light! It looked like the horizontal ends were capped by white glowing light bulbs! I was so stunned that I didn't even think to grab my cell phone to snap a picture!

This cross has never, ever looked like that before. Then when I looked at it a few minutes later, it looked like it always did, a dark bronzish brown or black, depending on the time of day and how the light hit it.

I must have seen that cross thousands of times at all hours of the morning, noon and night, and I have never seen anything like what I just described!

That afternoon, I decided to take a walk on the beach even though it was a cold, dreary day for Southern California.

The beach was quite deserted because of the grey and chilly weather. As I came to the end of the path on the sand where I usually turn around because of a creek that blocks my path, I noticed a jogger coming towards me from the creek.

He was jogging at a pretty good pace and he just kept going while I myself decided to turn around and go back. He did not stop.

Within less than a minute, on the same path that I had just walked, I noticed a large cross, deeply and perfectly drawn in the sand. It was definitely not there a minute ago!

It looked almost as if it was stamped into the sand because it was so perfect and straight. I thought, "wow, how interesting and unusual!" I stopped to look at it for a few seconds. I know that there was no one there walking behind me when I came to the creek where I turn around. Then, a few feet further in front of that cross were about ten others. Four were vertical, two were horizontal and four more were vertical! They all together looked like a huge Cross. They again were evenly spaced and perfectly carved in the sand.

But how?!!!

There was no one on that beach with me except for the jogger who did not stop.

I was very aware of his movements because I was quite alone out there.

Three cross experiences, three moon visions around the cross that faces my Healing table, three Miraculous visions of the sun caught on video, three people telling me that they see The Blessed Mother with me, three dolphins, three whale experiences, three rainbows, and on and on. . . .

Three signifies the Holy Trinity: God our Father, Jesus, His Son, and the Holy Spirit here on earth.

I have been Divinely Blessed to have been given this Sacred Gift of Healing and to have experienced all of these Amazing experiences along the way.

It has been a Sacred honor and privilege to be called to travel on this truly Amazing Journey with The Divine!

EPILOGUE

"I in them and you in me, that they may become perfectly one, so that the world may know that you sent me and loved them even as you loved me." (John 17:23)

BECAUSE YOU LOVED ME!

(Lyrics written by Diane Warren)

For all those times, You stood by me

For all the truth that You made me see

For all the joy, You brought to my life

For all the wrong that You made right

For every dream, You made come true

For all the love, I found in You

I'll be forever thankful

You're the One who held me up

Never let me fall

You're the One who saw me through it all

You were my strength when I was weak

You were my voice when I couldn't speak

You were my eyes when I couldn't see

You saw the best there was in me

Lifted me up when I couldn't reach

You gave me faith 'coz You believed

I'm everything I am

Because You loved me

You gave me wings and made me fly

You touched my hand I could touch the sky

I lost my faith, You gave it back to me

'You said no star was out of reach

You stood by me and I stood tall

I had Your love I had it all

I'm grateful for each day You gave me

Maybe I don't know that much

But I know this much is true

I was Blessed because I was loved by You

You were always there for me

The tender wind that carried me

A Light in the dark shining Your love into my life

You've been my inspiration

Through the lies You were the Truth

My world is a better place because of You

I'm everything I am

> *Because You loved me*

I'm everything I am

> *Because You loved me.*

A huge heartfelt thank you to God, "The Divine One," His Divine Son Jesus, Mother Mary, the Angels, the Saints, Mother Kwan Yin and the other Ascended Masters, my Spirit and Reiki Guides, and to all the other wonderful Divine Souls in Heaven and on earth who loved me!

With gratitude and Love!

ABOUT THE AUTHOR

Beverly is a Master Reiki Healer who lives and loves a very peaceful life on the ocean.

She connects best with God's Energy there.

The sun energizes her, the waves soothe her, and the sand grounds her. The dolphins and whales delight her.

She is watched over by God, Jesus, The Blessed Mother Mary, God's Angels, and other Divine Beings, as symbolized by Jesus's Cross that directly overlooks her Healing table.

She has had the great privilege of bringing a wonderful son into this world, who researches cures for diseases like cancer and AIDS, to name just a few.

He is also a Healer in his very own wonderful way. He is one of the great gifts bestowed upon her by The Divine.

In addition, God has Blessed her and her family with a beautiful grandchild.

She also feels very fortunate and grateful to have a husband who had agreed to move down to her favorite ocean town where she really finds her true peace and joy and who is also a very good sport about relocating for a while during her Healing Sessions.

She can be reached on Facebook at Master Reiki Healer:

https://www.facebook.com/Master-Reiki-Healer-1569284036713349

or via email at bev.pokorski@gmail.com.

ACKNOWLEDGMENTS

To God first and foremost.

Thank You for my life and all the wonderful Blessings that You have bestowed upon me . . . Your Holy Spirit, Your Son Jesus, His Mother Mary, the Angels, Ascended Masters, Saints and Guides, The Gift of Healing, my family, my friends, my health, my healing ocean . . . they are all truly priceless.

Thank You our dear Jesus for saving my life and guiding me along this Amazing Journey.

Thank You our dear Blessed Mother Mary for walking beside me and helping me fight the good fight.

Thank You for the Miraculous Visions of the sun and the moon.

Thank you to all of God's precious Angels, especially Archangel Raphael who brings God's Healing Energy to earth.

Thank you to Archangel Michael who fiercely protects us, gives us strength and courage and brings us calm so we can Heal.

Thank you, Archangel Galadriel and Archangel

Raguel, for strengthening my faith.

Thank you, Archangel Metatron for your protection.

Thank you, Archangel Gabriel for your messages and discernments.

Thank you, Archangel Melchizedek, for removing karmic trauma and for your esoteric wisdom.

Thank You God, Jesus, Blessed Mother Mary, Mother Kwan Yin and all the other Ascended Masters, the Saints and all of God's Angels and Divine Beings for the Magnificent Healing Miracles!

Thank you to all the pioneers that have gone before. It is often said that the pioneers take the arrows. Their courage and dedication have paved the way for a brave New World in Healing.

This has made it easier for our current generation of Light Workers to carry on with their calling. My hope is that we can accomplish in a big way what we came here to do.

Thank you to my special family. They are beautiful souls and very good sports who may not fully understand what I do or how it's done, but who were always there for me to practice my Healing skills on and to cheer me on.

Thank you to my very dear brother Rick, my only sibling, whose love, advice and support mean the world to me.

Thank you to my oldest and dearest best friend Melanie, whose love, advice, encouragement, support, and faith in what I do also mean the world to me.

Thank you to my dear soul friend Sheri, whose invaluable insights, advice, and support have always helped me tremendously along this Amazing Journey.

Thank you to my newest, dear soul friend Deanna, whose intuitive insights and wise advice have kept me focused on the sharing of my Journey. Thank you also for your tireless editing advice and dedication to this very special project. You have been a true treasure from the very first day we met.

Thank you to all those beautiful souls who entrusted their Healing to me and brought such joy into my world as I witnessed the Wonder of The Divine.

And thank you to all of my special earth Angels who would somehow mysteriously appear, (usually at the water, as when an unknown, special messenger just randomly approached me last summer to give me insight and more importantly, to inform me that The Blessed Mother was with me) when I needed them the most, ready and willing to help with their love, advice, guidance and support.

A very special thank you to Louisa Mastromarino, who channeled Jesus and the Blessed Mother for me and my client during my work on my breast cancer client with internal lymph node cancer.

Louisa was also my very own special earth Angel who facilitated my very own personal Miracles in Healing through God, Jesus, The Blessed Mother,

Mother Kwan Yin and other Ascended Masters, Angels and Saints. Thank you, many times, over!!!

She has also helped me to understand the significance of many of the Amazing experiences that I have encountered as I travel along my Journey with The Divine.

A very special thank you to my dearest earth Angel, Barbara Savin, who from the very beginning was always there for me and never once let me fall. She truly is one in a million! I do not know what I would have done without her!

May God Bless her and everyone that has shared my Amazing Journey with me along with those who grant me the privilege of sharing it with them through reading this book.

Thank you to all those kind and loving souls who have granted me permission to share their Healing experiences. Without them, this book could not have been possible.

www.ingramcontent.com/pod-product-compliance
Lightning Source LLC
Chambersburg PA
CBHW060859280326
41934CB00007B/1111